Ketogenic Diet Crash Course

Seriously Simple 7 Day Guide to Beating Cravings Whilst Turning Stubborn Fat into Energy

Robert M. Fleischer

Atlanta

ISBN 978-1-491284-13-1

9 781491 284131 >

All Rights Reserved

No part of this book may be reproduced or transmitted for resale or use by any party other than the individual purchaser who is the sole authorized user of this information. Purchaser is authorized to use any of the information in this publication for his or her own use only. All other reproduction or transmission, or any form or by any means, electronic or mechanical, including photocopying, recording or by any informational storage or retrieval system, is prohibited without express written permission from the author.

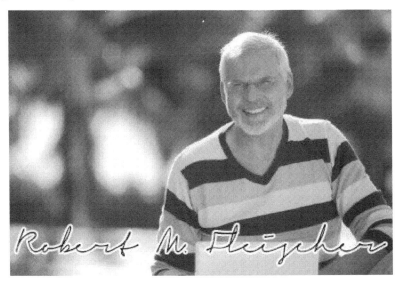

Copyright © 2012 Robert M. Fleischer

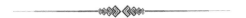

Testimonials

"I wish I had this book in college. I think life would have been a lot less painful then. Good job."

★★★★☆Donna Peters – Michigan

"Robert Fleischer cleared a lot of misconceptions I had about losing weight on a low carb diet. I now understand how to achieve sustained results."

★★★★☆**John R. Meyer – New York**

"I wasn't in the mood for another diet book, and this is another diet book, BUT this one got results for me and that's what matters. I'll never need another diet book ever again!"

★★★★★**Wendy Harrison – Santa Barbara**

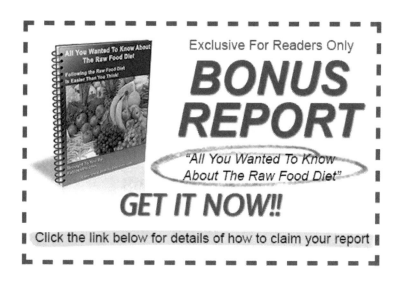

Exclusive Bonus Download: All You Wanted To Know About The Raw Food Diet

Raw food diets can be a great way to not only lose weight but also led a much healthier, natural lifestyle in general. Most raw food diets are plant-based, with at least 75% of the diet composed of raw food.

This short report will give you a bird's eye view about this all-natural diet plan!

You will learn:

- What is The Raw Food Diet Really Is!
- The Pros and Cons of the Rww Food Diet!
- Tools of the Trade!
- 7 Simple and Easy Raw Food Diet Meal Plans
- And MUCH MUCH MORE!

Download this guide and start improving your health NOW

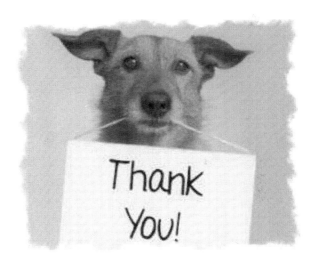

Thank you for downloading my book. Please REVIEW this book on Amazon. I need your feedback to make the next version better. Thank you so much!

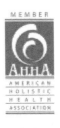

Books by Maggie Fitzgerald

The 7-Day Acid Reflux Diet

The 3-Step Diabetic Diet Plan

The Anti-Inflammatory Diet Plan

Ketogenic Diet Crash Course

Atkins Diet Beginners' Crash Course

www.amazon.com/author/robertfleischer

Is This Book for You?

A lot of people have been claiming for a long time that we live in a virtual world and today, more than ever, that seems to be the truth. There are smartphones, tablets and CCTV cameras everywhere. Wherever you are the chances are that someone is watching you. So in this virtual world of ours it is important to look good, and to feel good, otherwise things may stop going your way.

I wrote this book to help people understand how important a fit and healthy body is, and how obesity can destroy their lives. In order to have high self-esteem and project confidence someone has to look the part. If they are fat people will not take them as seriously as they should since in the majority's eyes looks go hand in hand with success.

These are hard times. We live in a cruel, competitive world in which everything can be seen as an advantage or a disadvantage. In order to survive in it people should do their best to look their best. My guide can help you achieve that goal, and, you know it's not as difficult as it sounds; all it takes is a decision and the will to work on it, and make some sacrifices along the way. It's simple as that.

TABLE OF CONTENTS

TESTIMONIALS 1

IS THIS BOOK FOR YOU? 4

AUTHOR'S INTRODUCTION 7

1. WHY GO ON A KETOGENIC DIET? 9

2. WEIGHT LOSS BASICS 15

3. KETO BASICS 19

    3.1. LOW-CARBOHYDRATE DIETS 19

    3.2. KETOSIS 21

    3.3. MACRONUTRIENTS IN THE KETOGENIC DIET 23

    3.4. A NOTE ON THE ATKINS DIET 25

4. THE KETOGENIC DIET 27

    4.1. TAILORING THE DIET TO YOUR NEEDS 34

    4.2. A NOTE ON OTHER TYPES OF KETOGENIC DIETS ... 38

5. EXERCISING TO MAXIMIZE WEIGHT LOSS 41

6. QUICK START GUIDE: 3 STEPS AND 7 DAYS TO A KETO DIET ... 51

7-DAY DELECTABLE RECIPES FOR MAXIMUM WEIGHT LOSS ... 53

BREAKFAST 53

    1. CHEESY BACON AND MUSHROOM QUICHE 53

    2. EGGS BENEDICT WITH SALMON 55

    3. ZUCCHINI AND BEEF BREAKFAST CASSEROLE 56

    4. ROSEMARY TURKEY MEATLOAF 58

    5. VEGGIE HAM OMELET 59

    6. NO-CRUST CHEESY SPINACH QUICHE 61

    7. TURKEY BREAKFAST SAUSAGE 62

LUNCH 65

    8. SPICY GRILLED SHRIMP 65

    9. ROASTED GARLIC-HERB PORK 66

    10. SALMON EGG SALAD 67

    11. BROCCOLI FISH BAKE 69

    12. GRAPE AND CHICKEN HOLIDAY SALAD 70

    13. SPICY TURKEY & VEGGIES STIR-FRY 71

14. SPINACH BEEF LOAF MUFFINS 73

DINNER **75**

15. HERBED CHICKEN CORDON BLEU 75
16. ASIAN BEEF LETTUCE WRAPS 76
17. HERBED PORK CHOPS OVER RASPBERRY SAUCE 78
18. CAJUN CHICKEN JAMBALAYA 79
19. SPINACH AND MUSHROOM STUFFED CHICKEN 81
20. HERB CRUSTED COD FILLETS 82
21. SPAGHETTI SQUASH WITH GARLIC MEAT SAUCE 84

DESSERT **87**

22. CHERRY CHEESECAKE BARS 87
23. CARROT BANANA MUFFINS 88
24. FRESH FRUIT SALAD WITH LEMON COCONUT CREAM 90
25. AVOCADO HAZELNUT MOUSSE 91
26. LOW CARB GRANOLA SNACK 92
27. CREAMY PEANUT BUTTER BALLS 93
28. MIXED BERRIES PARFAIT 94

EXCLUSIVE BONUS DOWNLOAD: ALL YOU WANTED TO KNOW ABOUT THE RAW FOOD DIET **97**

ONE LAST THING **99**

Disclaimer

While all attempts have been made to provide effective, verifiable information in this Book, neither the Author nor Publisher assumes any responsibility for errors, inaccuracies, or omissions. Any slights of people or organizations are unintentional.

This Book is not a source of medical information, and it should not be regarded as such. This publication is designed to provide accurate and authoritative information in regard to the subject matter covered. It is sold with the understanding that the publisher is not engaged in rendering a medical service. As with any medical advice, the reader is strongly encouraged to seek professional medical advice before taking action.

Author's Introduction

There is a huge need for this book right now. With the rise (and subsequent fall) of the Atkins diet, a lot of people have very serious misconceptions about low-carbohydrate and ketogenic diets. A lot of unsupported claims were made, then debunked, and a very reputable diet strategy was discredited. I'm writing this book to let you know that low-carb diets are not only safe, but can be very effective, and even healthy! Throughout my years of researching different diet strategies, this is one that I keep coming back to for various reasons. First of all, there's a lot of science behind it. Unfortunately, this science was disregarded by some high-profile people who supported ketogenic diets, much to their detriment. But, as you'll see, there are a lot of good reasons to revive low-carbohydrate diets. Second, keto diets (as they're called) can actually be a lot easier than other kinds of diets. Instead of severely restricting your calories, you cut your intake by a reasonable amount and make sure you're eating the right foods at the right times. Finally, the ketogenic diet is very adaptable, and can be modified for different needs, which is a huge bonus, and something that not a lot of other diets offer (chapter 4.1 goes into a bit more details on customizing your diet to your needs).

Of course, I'll be doing more than just defending the diet in this book. After laying out the basic principles of weight loss, I'll be explaining why keto diets are such a great way to lose weight in a safe, effective, and permanent way. And by combining the information in these two sections, I'll show you how to turn your body into a fat-burning machine that will have you at your goal weight in no time! And, finally, I've included a quick-start guide at the end of the book that condenses this information down into an easily readable form that you can keep around your house in case you forget exactly how many carbohydrates you're supposed to have, or which kinds, or when you're supposed to consume them. (This is also a great tool to share the basics of the ketogenic diet with others.)

I sincerely hope that this book makes a big impact on your weight loss efforts, and that you come to love the ketogenic diet as I have. It holds a very interesting place among other diets, and it has a lot of unique properties that you will come to know. The only thing that I ask of you before you start reading further is to keep an open mind. Like I said earlier, there are a lot of widely held misconceptions about this kind of diet. I'll do my best to debunk these myths, but you have to do your part as well, and not jump to conclusions! If you're willing to do that, I am confident that this book will show you how great the ketogenic diet is, and help you use it to get started on your way to your goal weight. Thanks for reading, and enjoy!

Sincerely,

Robert M. Fleischer

1. Why Go on a Ketogenic Diet?

Before answering the question of why you'd go on a ketogenic diet, I'd like to discuss the reasons why you might go on *any* diet. If you've been paying attention to the news over the past few years, you've probably been hearing about the "obesity epidemic." This is the term that's commonly used to describe the rapidly expanding waistlines of the American people. In 1994, when all 50 states began reporting obesity trends, a little less than half of the country was reporting 15–19% obesity rates. Ten years later, in 2004, only a handful of states were *under* the 15–19% block, while most states in the country stood at 20–24%, and an alarming 9 states reported over 25% obesity rates. In 2009, there was only a single state (Colorado) that was left in the 15–19% group, while about half of the country was in the 25–29% block, and 9 states showed over 30% obesity rates.[1] This is a huge increase in the incidence of obesity, and these statistics were only gathered over the course of fifteen years! If we don't stop this trend, we are going to see some very dire consequences, almost certainly within our own lifetimes.

So what's the big deal about obesity? Why is it something that we're working so hard to get rid of? In short, it's because obesity is linked with a huge number of other disorders that both lower the quality and shorten the length of life. On the quality side, obesity makes it more difficult to do a lot of things—playing with your kids, moving to a new house, going for a walk with your spouse, and maybe even just getting out to grab a drink with your friends. Being overweight means that you might experience reduced fitness, not have the strength to complete some daily activities, and get fatigued more easily; and none of these are fun things, especially when you're trying to keep up with the people around you. And when it comes to the life expectancy, obesity has even more significant effects. Having a body mass index (BMI) of over 30 has been linked to coronary heart disease, type 2 diabetes, high blood pressure, high cholesterol, bone disorders, and just about any other disease or condition that you can think of. The connections aren't always clear, but we can say with confidence that obesity makes you much more likely to contract a serious illness at some point in your life.

And that risk can be damaging to more than just your health—it can cost you a lot of money, too. You may have a great health insurance plan right now through your employer or you spouse's employer, but there's no guarantee that this will last over the next few months, let alone the next couple decades. There's been a lot of discussion about healthcare costs in the news over the past few years, and it's easy to see why: costs for appointment with family practice doctors can easily cost over $100, with visits to specialists getting into the $200s and above. And these are just for basic appointments. If you need tests, procedures, or referrals to other doctors, you're looking at additional expenses. And unless you're lucky enough to have an insurance policy that covers prescriptions, you'll likely be paying at least a co-pay for a large number of pills every month. And the expenses aren't just monetary—repeated visits to the doctor's office, procedures and prescriptions on a regular basis, and potential hospitalization for a serious condition take up a lot of time and effort, too. Wouldn't you rather spend this time doing something that you enjoy?

These costs don't just affect you, either—they can have a big impact on your family, especially if you have children. They'll spend more time taking care of you if you do contract a serious illness related to obesity. You won't be able to spend as much time with them doing what they love to do. And research has shown that children of obese parents are much more likely to be obese themselves, setting them up for the same problems that you might be experiencing in the very near future. I heard recently that children of two obese parents have an 80% chance of being obese themselves, while children of two non-obese parents have around a 10% chance. It's a big difference!

And there are more personal reasons, too. Many people want to lose weight so that they feel more attractive, and have more self-esteem and self-confidence. This is a really common reason for people to try to lose weight, and while there's no way to objectively measure the effects of weight loss on these things, it's easy to see why getting down to a "normal" weight range might be attractive for some people. Today's society places a huge value on being skinny and attractive—far too much value, in fact—but being trim, fit, and at a healthy weight is very attractive, and this is a goal that a very large number of people aim for when they start their weight loss process.

I've presented a very dire picture here, and you may think that I'm overstating the risks of being overweight. To be clear, most of the effects that I've listed above are much more likely, and likely to be worse in severity, for people who are obese than those who are overweight (keep reading to find out the difference and how to determine where you fall on the scale). Of course, if you're fifteen pounds overweight, there's less of a risk that you'll have these issues than if you're fifty pounds overweight. But there are risks at all levels, and your health is far too important to put on the line.

So why choose a ketogenic diet over the dozens (if not hundreds) of other options? If you're reading this book, it's likely that you already have at least some idea of why it's a good idea, but in case you just happened to pick up this book and flip to this page, I'll give a quick overview here. When it really comes down to it, there are three main reasons to choose a keto diet over any other type of diet.

1. To increase fat burning.

The main benefit of the ketogenic diet is that it improves your body's ability to burn fat. Your body generally uses stored carbohydrates as fuel when it can. This is an efficient process, but the effects are easily undone when you eat any more carbohydrates. What you really want to get rid of is *fat*. This is almost certainly why you're on a diet in the first place, and it's important not to lose sight of this benefit, because it's a big one that other diets just can't compete with. Your body uses a lot of calories, even when it's at rest, so if you can train it to use stored fat as a fuel instead of carbohydrates, you'll turn your body into a fat-burning machine. Not only this, but the high-protein foods that make up most of the diet increase your metabolism, meaning that you'll be burning even more calories without adding much activity to your daily schedule (although exercise is, of course, an important part of weight loss). The combination of boosting your metabolism and burning more calories from fat is a formidable combination that will have you lean in no time! And by turning fat into energy that your body can use, you're less likely be tired and irritable like you might be on other types of diets.

2. To avoid insulin resistance.

Insulin is one of the hormones that plays a huge role in weight management—it's released when you eat carbohydrates, and it modulates your metabolism and calorie storage. Proper insulin function is very important, because if it's not working properly, you end up with blood sugar that is far too high, a condition called hyperglycemia. Insulin resistance has been linked to many disorders, including type 2 diabetes, obesity, and a condition called "metabolic syndrome," which includes things like high blood pressure and bad cholesterol levels. Obviously insulin resistance is something that should be avoided! So how does it come about in the first place? Unfortunately, this isn't well understood. However, it does seem like high intake of carbohydrates, especially simple sugars, may play a role in increasing your body's resistance to the effects of insulin. I'll skip over a lot of the hard-to-understand science here; but to make a long story short, limiting the amount of carbohydrates that you consume makes sure that you retain your sensitivity to insulin, meaning that when you *do* consume carbohydrates, your body will process them efficiently and effectively. This is crucial in avoiding certain disorders as well as weight gain.

3. Eliminating harmful foods.

There's a lot of controversy in the food industry and medical field about where many of the diseases that are currently very common in the modern Western world come from. Truth be told, it's almost impossible to come up with a definitive answer, but an increasingly large number of people believe that a lot of them are linked very closely to our diet, and that carbohydrates are at least partly to blame. Let me be very clear about this: it's not that carbohydrates are inherently bad. They are, in fact, necessary for sustained bodily function. However, human beings are not well adapted to the levels of them that we currently consume. Our ancestors likely consumed very few carbohydrates, and the human body has not yet evolved to be better able to process different forms of carbohydrates (this is especially true of gluten). The results of this are as speculative as the cause, but increased inflammation, decreased hormone regulation, and digestive problems are a few of the things that are commonly attributed to the eating of too many carbohydrates—so drastically reducing the amount of carbs in your diet has obvious benefits. In addition to this, many of the processed and pre-packaged foods that have high concentrations of nasty chemicals, hormones, and pesticides are high in carbohydrates, and by avoiding these foods you'll be putting fewer harmful artificial substances into your body. On a more practical level, by eliminating things like artificial sweeteners and refined sugar from your diet, you'll help your body kick its addiction to sugar, which is something that can be very liberating when it comes to cravings.

There are more benefits to the diet than this, but I consider these to be the main three. As you read on, you'll discover many more reasons why ketogenic diets are not only effective for weight loss, but also very beneficial to your overall health. I know that you've probably heard a lot of bad things about low-carbohydrate diets, but keep an open mind, and I think you'll learn a lot of really good things!

2. Weight Loss Basics

Before getting into the details of the weight loss plan, I'd like to go over a few of the principles behind losing weight. A lot of this will be explained in more detail in the coming sections, but it's good to have at least a basic understanding of these concepts before getting into the plan itself. If you've been on a lot of diets before, or you're quite familiar with the principles behind weight loss, you can skip ahead to the next chapter on ketosis, but if this is the first time you've gone on a diet plan, I encourage you to read through the following points to increase your knowledge on diets and weight loss in general.

1. Calories.

When discussing dieting, we talk about calories all the time. But what is a calorie, really? A calorie is a unit of energy—to be exact, it's the amount of energy that's required to raise the temperature of one gram of water by one degree Celsius. When we talk about calories in food, what we're actually talking about is a kilocalorie, or one thousand calories, the amount of energy needed to raise a kilogram of water by one degree (having these two different definitions of the same term can be confusing, but you can be sure that every time calories are discussed in relation to food, it's actually a kilocalorie). When you understand that calories are used to measure energy, it's easy to see why they're so important, and why the body uses them in the way that it does. The body needs energy to keep functioning—your muscle use energy when they contract, even if it's just getting up from your chair or typing on a keyboard. Organs use energy when they perform necessary tasks like digestion, breathing, and the removal of toxins. Your body can extract needed energy either directly from food or from stored calories already in the body. Calories can be stored as a form of carbohydrate in the muscles, but it's generally stored as fat in various places in the body.

2. "Burning" calories.

When people talk about burning fat, what they're really talking about is mobilizing the calories that are stored in the body as fat. Every fat molecule that's stored in the body can be taken from its storage location (which can be anywhere, not just in your abdomen, thighs, and arms) and broken down by the liver, which releases other substances that are used by the body. These substances are then converted into energy to be used by muscles and organs. In this way, fat is converted into energy. And when does the body mobilize stored fat for energy? When it needs to use more energy than it can derive from carbohydrates that are currently available in the bloodstream or muscles. During exercise is the primary time that energy requirements are raised, which is one of the reasons why exercise is so important for weight loss. In short, it requires the mobilization of a lot of stored calories to fuel muscle movements.

3. Survival mode.

This is something that far too few diets take into account. Our bodies have evolved over time to be very good at storing calories, mostly because there were times when our ancestors didn't have enough food and had to rely on stored calories for energy. They also evolved a mechanism that's often called "survival mode," which is a reduction in metabolism when faced with a lack of food. What this means on a practical level is that when you're not consuming enough calories, your body actually undergoes some changes in its functioning to burn *less* and store *more* calories, which accomplishes the exact opposite of what you're trying to do with a diet. This is something to keep in mind when thinking about how many calories you should be consuming in a day. If you cut down too far, you'll be working against your body's natural functions, which is awfully inefficient.

4. Your ideal weight.

Deciding on your goal weight can be tough, and I highly recommend speaking with your physician or a qualified personal trainer to establish a good goal. However, as a starting point, you can use the body mass index (BMI), which is calculated as follows:

$$BMI = (\text{weight in lbs.}) / (\text{height in in.})2 \text{ x x } 703$$

You can also find a number of calculators online that will do this for you. Anyway, your BMI should be between 18.5 and 25. Between 25 and 30 is considered to be overweight, and over 30 is labeled as obese. No matter where you are on the scale, you *can* get down to the acceptable range. It may seem really far away, but trust me—you can do it!

Of course, there's a lot more to losing weight, especially if you start taking the biochemistry of it into account, but these are the most basic concepts that we'll be coming back to. If you're interested in learning more about these things, there's tons of free information available online that you can take advantage of.

3. Keto Basics

If you've decided to pick up this book, you likely already have an idea of what a ketogenic diet is and why you might consider using one. You might also already understand the benefits of sustained ketosis and how it can improve your life and take your weight loss and fat-burning to the next level. However, if someone gave you this book, or you just happened to pick it up because it sounded interesting, you might not know these things. This chapter is for you. But even if *do* already know a lot about the ketogenic diet, I encourage you to read the chapter anyway, because you're likely to learn something. There's a lot of false information out there regarding diets like this one, and it's important that we try to set the record straight on exactly how they work and why they're safe. And you're likely to get a lot of questions from people when you tell them you're on a keto diet—so you might as well read on to get the answers!

3.1. Low-Carbohydrate Diets

Many people believe that low-carbohydrate diets were invented in the 1970s, with Dr. Robert Atkins' diet system, called the Atkins Nutritional Approach. Others, however, believe that low-carbohydrate diets were first used in the 1920s as a treatment for epilepsy at the Mayo Clinic in a program headed by Dr. Mynie Peterman. While both of these systems were instrumental in bringing this kind of diet to the forefront of public consciousness, neither of them can be called "inventors" of the ketogenic diet. This kind of diet has actually been in use for far longer than this, with early mentions of fasting used to treat seizure disorders dating back to somewhere around 400 bc.[2] That's over two thousand years ago! This knowledge was passed down through the ages in various forms, primarily in medical circles, until it reached the interesting status that it holds today. You'll come to see that there are many different low-carbohydrate diet plans, but it's important to keep in mind that this is not a recent invention—these kinds of diets have been used successfully for a very long time.

So what defines a low-carbohydrate diet? There are a few different ways to answer this. First, it can be on a qualitative scale, meaning that you're on a low-carbohydrate diet when you've restricted your carbohydrates enough so that you're getting results, whether that's losing weight, building muscle, or just feeling better. There are no numbers associated with this, making it a hard system to follow. You just have to pay very close attention to how you're feeling and how many carbohydrates you're eating. The second is both more prescriptive and more quantitative—you aim for a certain number of carbohydrates every day. The number of carbohydrates varies by the diet, but it can be as low as 20 grams, and as high as 150 grams. This is a big range, and the number that you consume is often based on exactly what your goals are. This book is primarily about weight loss, so I'll be sticking with that as a goal.

What many people don't understand is that there's a point to a low-carbohydrate diet beyond just calorie restriction. Yes, by cutting out carbohydrates from your diet, you're likely to consume fewer calories throughout the day, and this is good when you're trying to lose weight. However, there's a more complicated physiological reason that low-carbohydrates work so well—this is a process called "ketosis," which will be discussed in the next section. For a very long time, ketosis wasn't fully understood, and people just stuck with low-carbohydrate diets because they worked. However, now that we have a more detailed understanding of this process, we can fully take advantage of it.

3.2. Ketosis

The word "ketosis" is often confused with "ketoacidosis," which is a wholly different thing. This section will detail the difference between the two and help you understand some of the science behind a ketogenic diet. We'll start with ketones: what are they? In a scientific sense, a ketone is any substance that belongs to a specific class of chemicals. In a nutritional sense, they're substances that are produced in the liver when fats are broken down. Ketones are stored in the body and they can be used as a fuel source for the body's activities, just as fat, protein, and carbohydrates can also be used for fuel. By far the largest store in the body is fat—if we could efficiently burn fat for fuel, our bodies would be able to sustain activity for very long periods of time. Unfortunately, our bodies are much better at using glucose, a sugar that is derived from carbohydrates—wouldn't it be great if we could teach our bodies to utilize fat instead of the glucose stored in carbs?

This is exactly what ketosis helps us do. When the production of ketones is accelerated, they start to build up in the blood, triggering the body to go into a state of ketosis. What this means on a practical level is that the body will now start using ketones for fuel instead of glucose. Most, but not all, systems in the body can use ketones for fuel. After staying in a state of ketosis for a few weeks, your body starts to adapt to this state, and nearly all of your muscles and organs will be using ketones instead of glucose for fuel; after further adaptation, however, your use of ketones will decrease, leading to an increase in the burning of fat. This is the primary goal of every ketogenic diet—the utilization of fat as the primary fuel in the body.

The body processes that lead to and follow ketosis are a bit complicated, but I'll try to present them here in a way that's understandable. We'll start with two hormones that are crucial in the process: insulin and glucagon. Insulin is a substance that is released in response to the consumption of glucose, and helps the body regulate its usage and the storage of carbohydrates. Glucagon is, essentially, the opposite—levels rise when there isn't much glucose available, and this causes the body to mobilize its fat stores for use as fuel. Obviously, if you're trying to get rid of fat, you want to lower your levels of insulin and raise your levels of glucagon. This is accomplished through a low-carbohydrate diet—by keeping the amount of glucose in your body low, you decrease the amount of circulating insulin, which increases your usage of glucagon.

Still with me? Now we'll go to the next step, the liver. The liver is a metabolic powerhouse, and plays a big role in determining whether you're in a carbohydrate-using or fat-using state. When the carbohydrate stores in the liver are exhausted, it triggers a drop in insulin and a rise in glucagon. When fats are used for fuel, they are broken down by the liver, and this process creates and releases ketones, increasing their concentration in the bloodstream. Normally, ketones are not used as a significant source of fuel for the body. However, the body will use whichever fuels are available, and by significantly raising the levels of ketones in the blood, you encourage your body to start using ketones instead of carbohydrates for energy. As I mentioned earlier, after some adaptation, most muscles and organs will stop using ketones for fuel, at which point your body begins utilizing the most efficient fuel source that's still available to it—fat. Once you've reached this state, your body will be deriving a large percentage of its total energy directly from fat stores. However, whether your body is using ketones or fat for fuel, it still requires the breakdown of fat stores by the liver, so the use of both of these sources can generally be considered a single process.

At this point, your body has become very good at using ketones and fat for fuels, which causes a decrease in the number of carbohydrates that you need, which further reduces the amount of insulin in circulation and—you guessed it—increases glucagon and keeps the process going. As you can see, the process of ketogenesis involves some pretty complex biochemistry. Fortunately, you don't have to totally understand it to take advantage of it. It can be beneficial to know what's going on, though, to make sure that you're adjusting your diet correctly at the proper times.

Ketoacidosis is, essentially, ketosis run wild. When the concentration of ketones in the blood gets too high, it can alter the pH of the body, which causes a lot of problems, and can actually be fatal if not treated. Don't worry, though—a ketoacidic state is quite difficult to achieve on a properly monitored and planned ketogenic diet. Most of the time, people who experience ketoacidosis are diabetic, on an extremely low-calorie diet, or drink heavily. All of these states can result in a significant increase in the amount of ketones in the blood that the body cannot handle. Some people believe that ketoacidosis is linked to low-carbohydrate diets, but by sticking to the plan outlined later in the book, you should have absolutely no problem avoiding it. It's important to remember (especially because you're likely to defend your diet against a few critics at some point or another) that ketoacidosis is generally brought about by underlying causes, such as diabetes or very high alcohol intake.

3.3. Macronutrients in the ketogenic diet

When it comes to nutrients that the body needs, there are two types: macronutrients and micronutrients. Macronutrients ("macro" means "large") are protein, carbohydrates, and fat. All of these are important, and each serves a different function. I'll outline the function of all of them here so that you understand why you can safely cut out carbohydrates from your diet. After all, you've been told to eat a balanced diet since you were in grade school—so why would you stop now? It's time to look at this advice more closely.

1. Protein.

This is a hugely important nutrient for your body—not only is it used for the creation of new cells and tissues, but it's also required for the repair of older ones. The cells in your body are constantly in a state of being replaced, and having enough protein allows this to happen normally—everyday life places a lot of wear and tear on our bodies, and protein is what lets us keep it going. Our need for protein is increased during times of growth or stress, like a workout—this is why children, adolescents, and athletes need more protein on a regular basis.

Protein is also used for energy, and confers 4 calories per gram. In cases of severe calorie restriction, the body will begin to catabolize (destroy for energy) muscles to get more protein to use as fuel, which is hugely detrimental to weight loss efforts. This is one of the grave mistakes that many people make when they go on diets, not realizing that they're actually damaging their bodies and hampering their efforts.

2. Carbohydrates.

Although I am advocating a low-carbohydrate diet in this book, it's important to understand that I'm not pushing for a *carbohydrate-free* one. Carbs, like protein, are needed—in fact, a small number of the body's systems cannot be fueled by ketones, and require carbohydrate for continued function. Because of this, you can't cut out every carbohydrate from your diet and expect things to go well. As I've mentioned before, carbs are a very readily available fuel for the body, meaning that when it needs energy, it goes to stored carbohydrates first (like protein, carbs have 4 calories per gram). While it's true that you're trying to train your body to use as much stored fat as possible, you still need to be able to access some carbohydrate stores when you're exercising, which is why the targeted and cyclical ketogenic diets (detailed in chapter 4.2) are popular among athletes.

So carbohydrates are important . . . but there are also some downsides. A prominent one that is they're easily stored as fat, and that consuming more than you need usually results in quick storage and weight gain. Another one is that they're very easy to eat a lot of, especially when you're eating low-quality ones, which will leave you feeling hungry again very quickly. This is an unfortunate cycle that results in increased carbohydrate intake and weight gain. And this increased intake can also lead to insulin resistance, which causes you to eat even *more* carbohydrates. As you can see, this is a vicious circle that is very difficult to get out of.

3. Fats.

During the low-fat diet craze, all fats got labeled as "bad," regardless of their composition or effects. This is extremely frustrating when you understand that it isn't fats that are the problem at all, but overeating! Fats are more efficient sources of energy than both protein and carbohydrates, as they have 9 calories per gram. They are also required for many important processes, including both immune and nervous system function. Although I'm championing this diet as a fat-burning one, it's with full knowledge that fats are very important, and that a certain amount of stored fat is crucial for overall well-being. Certain fats also have other benefits, like improving your blood cholesterol and reducing inflammation, which is one of the lesser-known causes of both obesity and a large number of other problems.

You've probably heard that fat is bad thousands of times over the past couple decades, but that's an idea that you have to get rid of right now. The problem is not with fat itself, but with how much of it, and what kind is consumed. I'll get into the differences later but for now, just know that you can maintain a healthy weight even when you're eating more fat than is usually recommended by a lot of diets—what's important is that you don't consume way too many calories, be they from fat, protein, or carbohydrates.

3.4. A Note on the Atkins Diet

When most people think of low-carbohydrate diets, they immediately think of the Atkins diet. This is both a blessing and a curse to those of us who are fans of ketogenic diets. The Atkins diet was—and still is—one of the most popular fad diets, and it's helped a huge number of people lose a lot of weight over the years. Unfortunately, it also caused a lot of health problems, too. I'd like to take a moment to talk about why this is and why you don't have to worry that the same things will happen on this diet.

The most significant difference between what Dr. Atkins recommended and the plan that I'm outlining here lies in calorie counting. Dr. Atkins believed that if people cut out most of the carbohydrates from their diet, they could eat high-protein, high-fat foods until they were full and still lose weight. And with some people, that's true—however, that's a rare blessing. Counting calories is one of the things that it just necessary to lose weight in a controlled and sustainable manner. If you're eating too many calories, it doesn't matter if they aren't coming from carbohydrates. Yes, your body is in a state of ketosis, and your insulin is well-managed, but if you consume more calories than you burn, you'll gain weight. Period. So the claim that you can eat as much as you want, as long as it's not carbohydrates, is very misleading. Don't be tempted to fall into this trap if you're going to start a ketogenic diet!

The Atkins diet was also problematic in that it didn't provide much guidance for when to consume carbohydrates or the best types to consume. As I mentioned before, carbohydrates are necessary, and it's important that your intake optimizes your body's use of them. This wasn't pointed out in the Atkins Nutritional Approach, and many people, thinking they could just cut out carbs either completely or very nearly so, didn't plan this part of their diet correctly, which resulted in problems.

4. The Ketogenic Diet

Now that you understand what ketosis is, how a ketogenic diet encourages your body to enter this state, and what the benefits are of dieting in this manner, you're probably anxious to get started! To help you start planning your diet, this section will present some general guidelines for maintaining a ketogenic diet. The following section will help you tailor these recommendations to your specific needs, ensuring that you're able to get into and maintain a state of ketosis on the diet.

1. Carbohydrate intake.

The first question that's always asked about low-carbohydrate diets is "How many carbohydrates should I be eating?" Of course, there are various answers to this, and different authorities and experts give different recommendations. Generally, you can attain a state of ketosis if you're consuming less than 100 grams of carbohydrates per day. However, this will raise the levels of ketones in your blood pretty slowly. To make sure that your fat stores are being mobilized at an adequate rate, I recommend aiming for 30 grams or less of carbohydrates each day. As an example, the following foods contain around 15 grams of carbohydrates:

- a slice of bread;
- 1/3 cup of cooked rice or pasta;
- 1/2 cup of beans
- 3 cups of popcorn
- 1 small piece of fresh fruit
- 1/2 cup of vegetables

So two servings of the foods above in a day would satisfy your requirement of 30 grams. If you can keep your carbohydrate intake at this level, you should reach a state of satisfactory and effective ketosis within the first couple weeks of the diet (though everyone goes through this process differently). Some people will take this piece of advice to mean that if you completely cut out carbohydrates, you'll achieve a state of ketosis more quickly. And while this is, in some ways, true, it's not recommended. Cutting anything completely out of your diet without the direct supervision of a physician isn't a good idea. As we saw before, this was one of the things that caused the demise of the Atkins diet. Not only that, but it's really hard to have a carbohydrate-free diet. A lot harder than you might think. So aim for 30 grams or so. You can increase your intake a bit later in the diet, but try to get under 30 grams daily for the first three to four weeks.

Simply restricting the number of carbohydrates that you consume is enough to get you into ketosis, but there are other strategies that you can also use to make sure that your insulin levels stay low. The first strategy has to do with the types of carbohydrates that you consume. Certain carbohydrates raise blood sugar (and, therefore, insulin) levels much more quickly than others. This is measured by the glycemic index (GI), a scale that is often used by dieters to help them choose foods that will keep them fueled and energized for longer periods of time. Things that are high on the scale, like white bread, white rice, some fruits, rice cakes, and table sugar, will raise your blood sugar very quickly. Foods that are lower on the index, including whole grains, most vegetables, nuts, seeds, and many beans give you a much more steady rise in blood sugar, preventing fat-storing insulin spikes. As you can see, the foods low on the scale have some things in common: namely, that they're high in fiber, protein, and fat. By choosing high-fiber options for your carbohydrate intake, you can help keep your body in a state of ketosis. Fortunately for those of us on low-carbohydrate diets, the GI values of meals are affected by all of the foods that are included in that meal, meaning that the protein and fat that you consume at the same time as carbohydrates will lower the GI value of the carbohydrate.

The final strategy you can take to keep your insulin levels low is to time your carbohydrate intake correctly. This isn't always easy, and depends a lot on your personal preferences, meal schedule, and how convenient something like this is for you. By spreading out your carbohydrate intake throughout the day, you can help make sure that blood sugar increases after meals are kept to a minimum. It can be hard to spread out 30 grams of carbohydrate over an entire day, as 5 or 10 grams of carbohydrates isn't very much. However, splitting up your intake into three phases of 10 grams or even two phases of 15 grams will help in this respect. Some people like to have all of their daily carbohydrates with one meal, and this is alright, too. But ideally, you should be splitting up the intake.

One final note here: alcohol is *very* detrimental to a ketogenic diet. Partly because a lot of alcoholic products contain carbohydrates (and more calories than you might realize), and partly because alcohol can prevent the body from going into a state of ketosis. I know that totally cutting it out of your diet may not be realistic, but try to at least minimize it as much as possible.

2. Protein intake.

Okay, so you're going to be drastically reducing the carbohydrates that you're ingesting, meaning that you'll have to increase your protein and fat intake to make sure you're getting enough calories in a day. How do you go about doing that? Is it safe? Are there certain types of proteins and fats that are best? We'll start with protein. Because having too little protein will leave you without enough calories, and too much will prevent ketosis (since your body will start burning the calories in the excess protein first, instead of converting fat into ketones like we want), it's important to get this in the right range. The best way to estimate how much protein you need is to use one of the following two equations:

Sedentary: 0.8 x bodyweight (lbs.)

Active: 0.9 x bodyweight (lbs.)

Convert the result of this equation into grams, and you have your protein requirement. For example, a 190-pound sedentary person would require 152 grams of protein per day (0.8 x 190 = 152). If this equation gives you a value of less than 150 grams, you should round up and have 150 grams of protein each day for the first three weeks of the diet. Consuming less than this, even if you're on the smaller side, can be detrimental to your weight loss efforts and your health. The difference between the sedentary and active levels has to do with both increased calorie requirements and increased protein requirements related to maintaining muscle mass, so don't be tempted to choose the sedentary equation if you exercise on a regular basis.

When your diet is largely made up of protein, it's important that you choose high-quality proteins that will provide you with the nutrients that you need to use it effectively. This means you should be eating a lot of meat, eggs, and dairy products, which contain complex proteins that provide the body with the different amino acids that it needs (amino acids are the molecules that protein is made of). Lower-quality proteins, like collagen and gelatin, are often found in things like low-quality protein shakes. You should avoid these in favor of high-quality ones, so if you're going to be having something like a protein shake or an energy bar, look at the list of ingredients to make sure that it includes high-quality animal proteins.

Getting a lot of protein is especially important in the first three weeks of a ketogenic diet, while ketogenic adaptations are still taking place. Once you've made it past the first three weeks of your diet, you can decrease your protein intake if you feel like you're getting too much. Above, I said that if you use the equations I provided and get a result of less than 150 grams per day, you should adjust up to 150.

After the first three weeks, this isn't the case—you can just use the equations to see how many grams you need.

3. Fat intake.

Just as you need to optimize your protein intake, you also need to think carefully about your fat intake to make sure that your ketogenic diet is a successful one. Before going into how many grams you need each day and other practical concerns, I'll be discussing the different types of fats. There are three main types: saturated, unsaturated, and trans-fats.

First, the difference between saturated and unsaturated fats. This is something that often isn't correctly understood. Saturated fats are often considered to be "bad" fats, but few people understand how they actually differ from unsaturated fats. Fats are classified based on the chemical structure of the molecules of which they're made up. To make a long story short, whether a fat molecule is saturated or unsaturated depends on how many hydrogen atoms are contained in the molecule. Saturated fats are found in animal products, like meat, eggs, milk, and cheese. Because of the high reliance of the ketogenic diet on high-protein foods, you're likely going to be consuming at least a moderate amount of saturated fat. This makes a lot of people nervous, as saturated fats have been linked to atherosclerosis and other cardiovascular diseases. However, the ketogenic diet allows the body to burn a huge amount of fat in a day, meaning that saturated fats won't be circulating in your body for very long. This is one of the reasons that a higher-than-normal fat intake on a ketogenic diet is advisable. In addition to this, I recommend some sources of beneficial saturated fats below, and by adding these to your diet, you'll help optimize your fat intake for both fat burning and overall health.

Unsaturated fats, on the other hand, come primarily from plant sources. These are generally considered to be healthier, and most diets recommend consuming primarily unsaturated fats. Because so many plant sources are high in carbohydrates, it can be difficult to balance unsaturated fat intake with carbohydrate avoidance. However, there are sources of unsaturated fats that can be used without

31

consuming too many carbohydrates. Oils, like those derived from olive and flax, are high in unsaturated fats, yet still low in carbohydrates. This makes them ideal for consuming on a ketogenic diet. It should also be noted that unsaturated fats include some essential fatty acids, including one that you've probably heard of: omega-3. Omega-3 is a fatty acid that helps reduce inflammation in the body, which will help both your weight loss and improve your overall health. Some of the best sources of omega-3 are oily fish (like salmon and mackerel), olive oil, and flax oil. Making sure to include these in your diet will be very beneficial on multiple levels.

The last type of fat, trans-fat, is a sub-type of unsaturated fat. Generally, trans-fats are created by the addition of hydrogen to an unsaturated fat—food manufacturers do this for a variety of reasons, but it's often to create a semi-solid texture (as with margarine, for example). Many people don't realize that trans-fats also occur naturally, in very small amounts, so they are something that our bodies can deal with, but man-made trans-fats are often found in very high amounts in processed foods, like packaged snacks, pre-prepared meals, and deep-fried foods (all of which you should avoid, especially on a diet). Trans-fats have been very strongly linked with a huge number of health issues, including coronary heart disease and other potentially fatal conditions. Many people blame it for the obesity epidemic, and a few have even made the claim that a very large number of modern, Western diseases can be traced to trans-fats. These fats came into fashion in the 1960s and 1970s when the food industry began to discourage the use of tropical oils, like coconut and palm oils. In general, you should be avoiding trans-fats at all costs.

Research has uncovered little evidence that fats are actually needed by the body, and a state of ketosis can be attained without fat intake. However, it's very difficult to get enough calories on a daily basis while only consuming protein and a small amount of carbohydrates. Because of this, I don't have any specific fat recommendations. As long as you're getting the right number of calories, consuming enough protein, and limiting your carbohydrate intake, the rest of your calories can come from fats. Just make sure that you're getting your fat from high-quality sources like extra virgin coconut, olive, and flax oil; cold-water fish; and other unprocessed foods.

4. Supplements.

The human body requires a huge number of different nutrients. Not only does it need the macronutrients—carbohydrates, protein, and fat—but it also requires a large number of micronutrients, a group of substances that includes things like vitamins and minerals. Here's a short list of a few examples with some of their main functions:

Vitamin B: used to regulate the body's use of energy.

Vitamin C: helps maintain proper immune function.

Iodine: used to create thyroid hormones.

Calcium: crucial for the creation and maintenance of strong bones.

Folate: important for successful pregnancy.

This list includes only five different vitamins and minerals, but you can see that they're important in a wide variety of processes that take place in the body. It's easy to understand why a deficiency in a single micronutrient can throw your body out of whack and cause some pretty serious problems, and it becomes obvious very quickly that getting enough of these substances is crucial not only for weight loss, but for general health and well-being. These micronutrients are found in a wide variety of different foods, which means that cutting a certain food group—like produce and bread products—out of your diet can cause problems if you don't make up for the micronutrients that you're no longer getting from these food sources. The best way to do this is through supplements. I recommend a high-quality multivitamin—not just one from the corner drugstore, but one from a health foods store where the staff can help you pick out the right supplement for you. Places like Whole Foods, Sprouts, GNC, the Vitamin Shoppe, and other similar stores are good places to find these high-quality supplements. If you know what you need, you can also find them online.

I also recommend taking both an anti-oxidant and a fish oil supplement. These will help to minimize damage done to your muscles through exercise and other processes as well as manage inflammation. Again, getting high-quality versions of these is important.

4.1. Tailoring the Diet to Your Needs

Because every body functions differently, everyone has different dietary needs, and this applies to diets as well. Any diet that claims to have a single solution for everyone should be regarded with suspicion! Below, I've outlined a few ways in which you can adapt the ketogenic diet plan to your specific body, situation, and goals.

1. The calorie deficit.

As discussed before, every diet is based around the same principle: establishing a calorie deficit. If you're eating more calories than you're burning, you'll gain weight. If you consume fewer calories than you use, you'll lose weight. There's no getting around this. Even on a ketogenic diet, where calorie-burning works a bit differently than in other diets, this is a rule that can't be broken if you're going to succeed in losing weight, and it's something that you have to get right. So let's take a look at how you should determine how many calories you'll need in a day.

The first thing that you'll have to figure out is your basal metabolic rate (BMR). This is the number of calories that your body burns in 24 hours when it's at rest. If you were to stay in bed all day, you'd still burn this many calories. This makes up a huge portion of the number of calories you burn in a day. There are a lot of different equations out there to estimate your BMR, but this is a good one:

Women: BMR = 655 + (4.35 x weight in pounds) + (4.7 x height in inches) - (4.7 x age in years)

Men: BMR = 66 + (6.23 x weight in pounds) + (12.7 x height in inches) - (6.8 x age in years)

This will give you a general idea of how many calories your body burns at a baseline rate. Of course, just like anything else, there's a lot of inter-individual variability. Because of this, you might want to consider having your BMR tested to get a more accurate measurement; if you'd like to get more information about this, talk to your doctor or a personal trainer at a health club, and they should be able to help get you tested. After determining your BMR, you have to take into account how many calories you burn through exercise. You can approximate this by multiplying your BMR by a factor depending on how active you are to get a total average calorie expenditure for a day (we'll call this the adjusted BMR"):

- If you are sedentary (little or no exercise), use BMR x 1.2
- If you are lightly active (light exercise or sports 1–3 days/week), use BMR x 1.375
- If you are moderately active (moderate exercise or sports 3–5 days/week), use BMR x 1.55
- If you are very active (hard exercise or sports 6–7 days a week), use BMR x 1.725
- If you are extra active (very hard exercise or sports, a physically demanding job, or training 2x/day), use BMR x 1.9

Once you've gotten your total for the day, all you have to do is consume fewer than that number and you'll start losing weight! A good goal is to establish a 500-calorie deficit each day of the week. This will lead to about a pound of weight loss each week, which is considered a safe amount to lose. Some people can lose more than this, especially in the beginning of their weight loss plans, but over an extended period of time, a pound each week is a sustainable, effective goal. This is true for every diet, including a ketogenic one.

Here's an example, just to make sure you fully understand how to calculate your calorie goal. Let's take a woman with the following statistics:

- Weight: 170 lbs.
- Height: 5'7" (67 in.)
- Age: 42
- Exercise: light, twice a week.

Using the BMR equation, we get the following: 655 + (4.35 x 170) + (4.7 x 67) – (4.7 x 42) = 1512 x 1.375 = 2079. To establish a 500-calorie deficit, this woman would have to consume approximately 1579 calories per day.

2. Practical concerns.

Just knowing that you need to establish a deficit isn't enough—you actually have to do it! Which means that you'll be counting calories. After a few weeks, you'll likely have adjusted to your new daily caloric intake, and you'll be in a state of ketosis, so you might be able to stop counting. But for the first several weeks, I strongly recommend it. There are two different ways you can go about this. The first method, which is the one that I prefer and have used in the past, is to track your calories by using an online service like LoseIt! or MyFitnessPal. These are free services that allow you to enter the foods that you eat and see what your caloric intake for the day is. LoseIt! allows you to include recipes as well, which is very useful if you eat the same dish often, and a previous meals option that allows you to copy a meal from sometime in the last week into the current day. There's a database full of foods that already have nutrition information, and you can enter custom items for anything that's not already in the database. You can also get apps for both of these services on iOS or Android, which makes it easy to remember to update your food log.

Of course, you might find that keeping an old-fashioned notebook-based food journal is best for you. This is the second option, and some people find that they like it more or that they're motivated to do it. If you decide to use the paper method, you'll have to look up the nutrition information for every food that you put into your log, so you might be spending more time on this part of the diet. Many people find, however, that just writing down what they eat, even without the specific nutritional information, is motivating enough to get them to reduce their caloric intake to maintain a calorie deficit. Feel free to try both the electronic and paper methods, but make sure that you stick to your plan.

3. Eating for exercise.

Exercise is an important part of any weight-loss strategy, as it adds to the calorie-burning side of the caloric equation (I find that exercise is usually the main part of my weight-loss efforts, in fact, because it allows me to eat more while still maintaining a deficit!). Because your body is using more energy, it will burn more fuel—this also means, however, that it requires more fuel. This is why exercising often makes you hungry. And if you're not getting enough calories, it'll be really hard to exercise. So you'll have to balance your increased caloric needs with the need to maintain a deficit. Using one of many online services that will tell you how many calories that you burn in a certain amount of time spent doing a particular activity can be extremely helpful here (I like the one at bodybuilding.com/fun/calories.htm). Most of the calorie-logging websites and apps provide you with this information as well, and there are plenty of other resources online that you can use to get an estimate of how many calories you've burned. You should be eating as many calories as you're burning while keeping the rest of your diet 500 calories below your daily expenditure. For example, if your adjusted BMR is 1900, and you burn 400 calories on a run, you'll have a total expenditure of 2300 calories for a day. You can eat 1800 calories to maintain your 500-calorie deficit.

4.2. A Note on Other Types of Ketogenic Diets

Because glucose is generally the preferred fuel of the body for performing exercise, individuals who train at high intensities might have difficulty with the standard ketogenic diet that was detailed previously. Although a perpetual state of ketosis helps the body to burn fat, it doesn't always provide enough fuel for high-intensity workouts, such as those completed by weight lifters or endurance athletes. Even if you're not an elite athlete, you may find that working out while you're on a ketogenic diet is difficult. For this reason, two alternate methods of dieting have been devised, each of which aims to optimize carbohydrate intake to ensure the proper fueling of workouts. These are the cyclical ketogenic diet (CKD) and the targeted ketogenic diet (TKD), both of which will be discussed here.

Before outlining these plans, I'd like to note that not everyone who works out needs to use one of these plans. You should try the standard keto diet and see if you have problems exercising before attempting one of these, as they can be significantly harder to stick to.

1. The targeted ketogenic diet.

The premise of this variation on the standard keto diet is simple: consume some carbohydrates before a workout, both to give your body a little extra fuel during the training session and to help your body synthesize glycogen after the workout, setting you up for success in the next session. Although your body generally has enough fuel for training when you're in a state of ketosis, most people find it beneficial to have some carbohydrates before training, and this is a popular variation for people who exercise regularly. There are various formulas that can give you an estimate of how many grams of carbohydrate you should consume before your workout, but if you stick to the 25–50 gram range, you should find that training and recovery are easier. If you're completing a very large amount of high-intensity training (if you are, for example, a weight lifter or an elite endurance athlete), you may want to also have some carbohydrates during or after your workout as well—if you're burning enough calories throughout your workout to get through all of the glucose that you've ingested, this can be a good idea. No matter when you're consuming your carbohydrates, it's a good idea to stick to simple sugars and other high-GI foods.

Many people ask if a targeted keto diet will move their bodies out of ketosis during their workout. The answer, simply, is yes. Depending on how hard you're working, and how many grams of carbohydrate you're consuming, you might be out of ketosis for a very short time or a little longer, but the benefits of this type of diet greatly outweigh the drawbacks, especially if you're using a ketogenic diet to aid you in training for a sport or a specific event. Because you only ingest carbohydrates at specific, high-use times, you'll maintain your state of ketosis and burn through your fat stores quickly.

2. The cyclical ketogenic diet.

This diet is similar to the targeted keto diet above, but involves a bit more planning. Because this is slightly more difficult to do, and requires more detailed attention, it's usually used by serious athletes; in addition to the increased effort, it also requires that you burn through a lot of carbohydrates during training sessions, so it's less effective for maintaining a state of ketosis if you're not doing a lot of high-intensity workouts. The name of the diet comes from the cycling of ketogenic and high-carbohydrate days: generally, it's recommended to go 5–6 days on a normal ketogenic diet, and then have 1–2 days of high-carbohydrate eating. Both longer and shorter cycles have been tried with success, and using the 7-day week is generally a matter of convenience more than anything else. You can go anywhere from 3 to 12 days between your carb-loading days and still get the intended effects.

During the high-carbohydrate phase of the cycle, the goal is to get as much glycogen into your muscles as possible so that they're fully fueled for the next cycle of training. It's hard to know how many grams of carbohydrates are needed to replenish the glycogen in your muscles, and it depends a lot on how hard you're training during the ketogenic portion of the diet. If you're interested, you can find quite a few more detailed, scientific CKD plans online, and if you'd like to get a personalized recommendation for the cyclical keto diet, I encourage you to speak to a sports nutritionist, who can give you very specific figures to aim for.

I should also note that because this is a difficult diet to remain on, and because there aren't any long-term studies that provide insight into how it affects adaptation to ketosis, it's a good idea to use this sparingly, and only when you really need to ramp up your training for something, like an important competition.

5. Exercising to Maximize Weight Loss

Now that you understand how to go on a ketogenic diet, it's time to get a good idea of how you can use exercise to boost your fat burning and improve your body composition. Something that a lot of people don't understand is that to get the look you're after (which is usually a toned, trim, fit look), you don't need to just burn fat, but you also need to build a bit of muscle, too. This is one of the reasons that exercise is so important. Of course, there's more to it than aesthetics. Exercise also helps you burn a lot of calories, and has quite a few other health benefits, as well. I'd like to discuss some of these benefits before getting into the details of how you should be using exercise to supplement your ketogenic diet.

You've probably been told that "exercise is good for you" at least a thousand times, but how often does someone take the time to explain to you *why* it's good for you? Probably not very often. There have been entire books written on this topic, so I'll just give you a quick overview here.

1. Cardiovascular benefits.

Aerobic exercise taxes your heart, lungs, and circulatory system, meaning that they all get stronger over time. This is important because it helps you ward off cardiovascular disease, and this is especially if helpful if you're genetically predisposed to some sort of cardiovascular condition, like atherosclerosis or congestive heart failure. The preventative effects come about mainly through a reduction of your blood pressure and an improvement in your HDL-to-LDL cholesterol ratio (though there are other mechanisms as well).

Aerobic exercise may also improve the ability of your blood vessels to dilate when needed, which helps get oxygen to your muscles when they need it most. And, of course, performing regular exercise will improve your ability to complete daily tasks, like carrying things up the stairs, running around with your kids, and re-decorating, all of which can tax your cardiovascular system.

2. Musculoskeletal benefits.

Obviously, using your muscles on a regular basis makes them better able to handle the strain you put on them when you're exercising—put simply, you get stronger when you use your muscles regularly. This has all kinds of benefits in everyday life—think about if you were to go to the store right now and buy a new set of kitchenware. Would you be able to lift a box full of saucepans, frying pans, and stockpots? If not, you might be in need of some serious muscle-strengthening exercise. As people age, they tend to lose muscle mass (this is true of both men and women), and by building up your muscles before this starts happening, you'll be better able to continue doing your regular activities later into your life, which is something that everyone wants to do.

When you do weight-bearing exercise (like weightlifting, walking, running, and sports), your bones are faced with increased stress when your feet hit the ground, no matter whether it's from a single walking step or from landing after a jump shot on the basketball court. The stress placed on your bones causes them to strengthen, which is really important as we get older. This is especially true for women who are post-menopausal or close to it, as they are at increased risk of osteoporosis. By strengthening your bones before you're faced with a debilitating condition like this, you'll make it less likely that you'll go through the very unpleasant experience of breaking a bone sometime in your life.

3. Mental health benefits.

This is something that a lot of people don't mention in their discussions of exercise (or of dieting). I find that very unfortunate, because it's a *huge* benefit of exercise, and it can have a much larger

42

effect on your weight loss efforts than you might think. Although not everyone lists exercise as their favorite stress-busting activity, it's a pretty common one. Getting in 45 minutes on the elliptical, running for 30 minutes, swimming a half-mile, or biking out of town are great ways to release some of your pent-up stress. I find this to be especially true when you're outside, in nature, and you don't have the distractions of your smartphone, your laptop, or your kids. When you're working out, you can just let your mind wander, and this is when you have some of your best ideas, and when you have a lot of realizations that you just don't have time for during the rest of the day.

Why is stress relief so important for weight loss? This is a complicated topic, but what it comes down to is that stress and weight gain have a very strong relationship that is hormonal as well as habitual. Stress and eating go together in a huge number of people—whether you tend to eat more or eat less when you're stressed, you're getting away from your natural, healthy eating pattern, and that's not good for weight loss. Stress also releases cortisol, a hormone that, along with insulin, plays a role in fat storage, and increases fat storage in your abdomen, which is not only very unhealthy, but also pretty unsightly. So take my word for it—stress will be detrimental to your weight loss efforts. Exercise and get rid of some of it!

Okay, so now you have a good idea of why exercise is so important, not just as a supplement for your diet, but as a way to improve your general health. You probably have some questions about how you should be exercising and how much. Fortunately for you, I have some guidance related to this as well! Again, there have been huge books written about things like this, but I'll try to condense it down here so you get the basics.

1. Choose exercise that works for you.

I can't stress this point enough. A lot of people, when they find out that they should add exercise to their diet, force themselves into the gym to do whatever seems like the most effective calorie-burning exercise they can find, and they get burnt out really quick. They think they don't like exercising, but what they *really* don't like is the exercise that they've chosen! Trust me when I say that exercising just to burn calories is not the best way to go about it. It's important to find something that you really enjoy doing, or else it's going to be a struggle to motivate yourself to do it. If you don't already have an activity that you really like, I have a few suggestions.

First, just try walking. I know this doesn't sound like it will do much, but walking is actually a really great whole-body exercise that uses your large muscle groups, gets your heart rate up, and helps strengthen your bones. A brisk 30-minute walk is one of my favorite ways to get exercise, especially in the autumn, when the trees are turning red and orange—I love it! Some people like to take really long walks a few times a week, others enjoy quick walks a couple times a day—it's up to you. Just get out there and move.

Second, try something new: give tennis a shot, or throw a frisbee in the park, or join a community softball team. Take an aerobics class or start some weightlifting (if you're feeling quite athletic, try kettlebells or a class like BodyPump). Challenging yourself is a really fun way to both meet new people and get exercise. When I moved to a new city recently, I joined a mountain biking group, and I've met people and gotten to explore the surrounding area—it's definitely a great way to get to learn a new place. Try out a bunch of different things and see what you like! You never know what you might discover. For a very long time, I thought that I would never enjoy dancing, but my wife got me into swing dancing a few years ago, and it's become one of my favorite activities. (Lindy hop, by the way, is a fantastic and really fun way to exercise!)

Finally, make sure that you're continually challenging yourself. If you decide to pick up swimming, and you start with 15 minutes at a time, make sure to step it up to 20 minutes in a couple weeks. Then 30 minutes. Then 40. When your body adapts to a particular form of exercise, it's going to get a lot easier, which is a great feeling, but it also means that you're also not quite getting the same workout that you were. And when this happens, be proud of yourself! You're making a lot of progress. You may be on a diet, but don't forget to celebrate from time to time when you make a breakthrough. It's a really important part of exercising and marking your achievements.

2. Exercise the right amount.

"How much should I exercise?" has to be one of the most common questions I get when talking about losing weight. Usually it's asked with some trepidation, as people think that I'm going to tell them they need to exercise every day of the week. As with just about everything, it largely depends on your goals and how much you like to exercise. I could give you a long-winded explanation of what you should aim for, but I'll just give you this handy chart from the CDC instead:

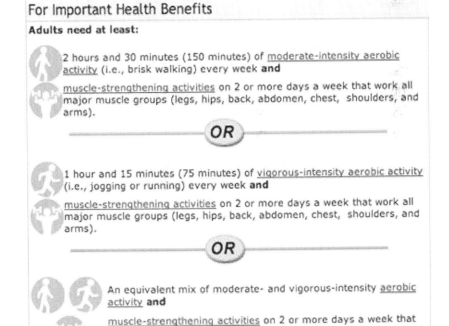

For Important Health Benefits

Adults need at least:

2 hours and 30 minutes (150 minutes) of moderate-intensity aerobic activity (i.e., brisk walking) every week **and**

muscle-strengthening activities on 2 or more days a week that work all major muscle groups (legs, hips, back, abdomen, chest, shoulders, and arms).

OR

1 hour and 15 minutes (75 minutes) of vigorous-intensity aerobic activity (i.e., jogging or running) every week **and**

muscle-strengthening activities on 2 or more days a week that work all major muscle groups (legs, hips, back, abdomen, chest, shoulders, and arms).

OR

An equivalent mix of moderate- and vigorous-intensity aerobic activity **and**

muscle-strengthening activities on 2 or more days a week that work all major muscle groups (legs, hips, back, abdomen, chest, shoulders, and arms).

For Even *Greater* Health Benefits

Adults should increase their activity to:

 5 hours (300 minutes) each week of <u>moderate-intensity aerobic activity</u> **and**

 <u>muscle-strengthening activities</u> on 2 or more days a week that work all major muscle groups (legs, hips, back, abdomen, chest, shoulders, and arms).

 OR

 2 hours and 30 minutes (150 minutes) each week of <u>vigrous-intensity aerobic activity</u> **and**

 <u>muscle-strengthening activities</u> on 2 or more days a week that work all major muscle groups (legs, hips, back, abdomen, chest, shoulders, and arms).

 OR

 An equivalent mix of moderate- and vigorous-intensity <u>aerobic activity</u> **and**

 <u>muscle-strengthening activities</u> on 2 or more days a week that work all major muscle groups (legs, hips, back, abdomen, chest, shoulders, and arms).

Obviously, for weight loss, you should be aiming for more, rather than less, exercise. You may notice that both moderate- and vigorous-level activities are included here. Which exercises fall into which category? The CDC recommends brisk walking, water aerobics, bike riding, playing doubles tennis, and pushing a lawn mower as activities that are at the moderate level. Vigorous activities are things like running, biking fast or on hills, swimming laps, and playing basketball, singles tennis, or other sports. In addition to aerobic exercise, you should also be doing muscle-strengthening activities, like lifting weights, using resistance bands, body-weight exercises, or yoga, twice a week. This might sound like a lot, but if you start with just a little bit and work your way up, you'll be there in no time! Don't worry if you can't just jump right into it—losing weight and gaining fitness are both long-term goals, so just focus on what you can do now, and try to get up to a little more each week.

3. Do some interval training.

When it comes to aerobic exercise, there's been a lot of discussion about the best forms of exercise for burning calories and improving body composition. Some people say that doing really long low-intensity workouts is the best way to go, as it burns fewer calories, but a higher percentage of those calories are from fat. Others say that very high-intensity workouts that completely drain you of energy are better, as they burn a huge amount of total calories. However, scientists are beginning to discover that a balance between the two is actually the most effective for burning calories and increasing fitness—this is the premise of interval training.

Interval training is a type of training that consists of a longer low-intensity workout interspersed with shorter high-intensity phases. For example, an interval workout done while running would look something like this:

- 10 minutes easy jog
- 5 minutes hard run
- 10 minutes easy jog
- 5 minutes very hard run
- 10 minutes easy jog
- 5 minutes hard run
- 10 minutes easy jog

Obviously, there are a lot of different ways to combine the different phases of the workout, and these types of training sessions can be tailored to your specific goals. You can do a form of interval training for a weight lifting workout, too, by using a treadmill or an exercise bike:

- 10 minutes exercise bike
- 3 sets of weight lifting
- 5 minutes exercise bike
- 3 sets of weight lifting
- 5 minutes exercise bike

- 3 sets of weight lifting
- 10 minutes exercise bike

Again, there are tons of different options that you can use for a workout like this. What's important is that you keep your heart rate up for an extended period of time and get a few high-intensity bouts in as well. I strongly encourage you to give this a try! I wouldn't recommend doing this kind of workout if you're just getting started with exercise, but if you're pretty comfortable with working out, it's a great way to try something new and torch a lot of calories. And trust me: you will really feel like you've accomplished something when you're done!

4. Make exercise a part of your life.

This absolutely cannot be overstated. Effective weight loss doesn't just require the adoption of a few new habits—it really needs a change in lifestyle. This is also true of becoming more fit. To really make exercise a part of your new lifestyle, you have to not just do it every once in a while, but to love it and to see opportunities to exercise everywhere. This is tough to teach, but there are a few steps that you can take to help yourself get to this stage. First, get an exercise partner and schedule your workout sessions in advance. We're awfully reliant on our electronic calendars today, and you can take advantage of this by getting your tennis date or your scheduled jog on your calendar. With most of these calendar products, you can even invite other people to them, meaning that you can make sure the same calendar event will be on you workout partner's schedule, too! It's pretty convenient.

Second, make the choice to work exercise into your life every chance you get. Have the chance to take the elevator or escalator? Take the stairs instead. Tempted to drive around the parking lot looking for a spot close to the door? Park farther away and walk. Just need milk and eggs from the grocery store? Don't drive—ride your bike or walk and bring a backpack. It's things like this that burn just a few extra calories, but add up to a big expenditure over time. If all of this sounds like a lot of extra work, you can get frequent exercise in other ways. If you work at a desk, stand up and stretch every 15 minutes, and go for a 10-minute walk twice during the weekday. You'll be doing your body a favor!

Finally, always have a fitness goal in mind. I find this to be extremely helpful. It should be separate from your weight-loss goal, and you should be able to achieve it in a shorter amount of time. This is great for motivation, as you'll always feel like you're approaching your goal, even if you're still 20 pounds away from your goal weight. For example, if you can run 4 miles in 45 minutes right now, make it a goal to run 4 miles in 40 minutes. Or 5 miles in 50 minutes. If you can currently do three sets of squats with 60 pounds, aim for three sets with 80 pounds. It can also be a skill-based goal, like learning to do an overhand serve in tennis or to shoot a three-pointer in basketball. No matter how you're getting your exercise, set a goal. It's more fun, more rewarding, and more motivating!

6. Quick Start Guide: 3 Steps and 7 Days to a Keto Diet

This quick start guide will get you from your current diet to a ketogenic one in 7 days. While reading the rest of this book is important, if you have to condense it down to one page for someone else, this is the page!

Step 1 (days 1–2): stock your cupboards for success.

If you're going to cut back on carbohydrates, you'll need something to replace them with! By replacing them with protein and fat from healthy sources, you'll ensure that you're not missing out on the nutrients your body needs to function properly. What are healthy sources? Natural and organic meats, oily fish, eggs, dairy products, and oils, like extra virgin coconut and olive oils. You'll also want nuts and seeds for snacks. Don't get rid of every source of carbohydrates in your house, though—you'll need to keep a few around to get your daily intake. Items that are low on the glycemic index, like green leafy vegetables, whole grains, beans, and hummus are good.

Step 2 (days 3–5): start tapering off of carbs.

Going from a normal diet to a ketogenic one without preparing your body is really tough, and I don't recommend it. These three days will help your body adapt to your new caloric intake before going into the standard low-carbohydrate phase. On day 3, aim for about 100 grams of carbohydrates; on day 4, aim for 75 grams; on day 5, 50 grams. This will help your body ramp up its fat-burning metabolism and prepare to process all of the protein and fat that will be making up most of your caloric intake on the keto diet.

Step 3: (days 6–7): complete the carbohydrate taper.

Your carbohydrate intake on the final two days of this week should be at the level that you'll be aiming for in the first phase of the diet, as discussed in chapter 4. Do your best on these two days to get under 30 grams per day (and, if you can, split your intake between two or three different meals throughout the day). I include these days here, instead of as the first part of the diet, in case you have trouble making it down to 30 grams. If you can't quite get there, that's okay. This is your preparation week, and the diet hasn't actually started yet, so you'll have a better idea of what you're getting yourself into. It's a great way to practice and see if any issues come up. You might find that you have some food sensitivities that you weren't aware of, or you could discover that you'll need more high-protein snacks. That's why these days are important!

Once you've gotten through the first week, you'll be on track to continue with your ketogenic diet! Stay under 30 grams of carbohydrates per day, and aim for at least 150 grams of protein each day for the first three weeks of the diet (to get more specific protein recommendations, see chapter 4). You're on your way to becoming an efficient fat-burning machine!

---

[1] This data was retrieved from the CDC's Overweight and Obesity webpage.

[2] I want to make this very clear as early as possible, just in case this statement is open to misinterpretation. This is not a fasting diet, and ketogenic diets do not require abstinence from food. However, the processes that the body undergoes when fasting are similar to the processes that are activated when on a low-carbohydrate diet, and this is why these kinds of diets are often discussed together.

7-Day Delectable Recipes for Maximum Weight Loss

Breakfast

1. Cheesy Bacon and Mushroom Quiche

Servings: 5
Preparation time: 10 minutes
Cook time: 50 minutes
Ready in: 1 hour

Nutrition Facts

Serving Size 206 g

Amount Per Serving

Calories 522   Calories from Fat 349

	% Daily Value*
Total Fat 38.7g	**60%**
Saturated Fat 16.9g	**85%**
Trans Fat 0.0g	
Cholesterol 220mg	**73%**
Sodium 990mg	**41%**
Total Carbohydrates 17.8g	**6%**
Dietary Fiber 0.8g	**3%**
Sugars 3.1g	
Protein 25.5g	

Vitamin A 19%	•	Vitamin C 16%
Calcium 33%	•	Iron 11%

Nutrition Grade B

* Based on a 2000 calorie diet

Ingredients

- 3 ounces nitrite/nitrate free bacon bits
- 1 cup sliced mushrooms
- 1/2 teaspoon fresh grated nutmeg
- 1/2 cup chopped onion
- 1/4 chopped red bell pepper
- 8 ounces shredded Italian cheese blend
- 1 (9 inch) deep dish frozen pie crust
- 4 eggs, lightly beaten
- 1 cup half-and-half cream

Directions

1. **Preheat** oven to 400 degrees F (200 degrees C). Line a 9-inch pie plate with the pie crust.
2. **Combine** the bacon, mushrooms, nutmeg, onions, bell pepper, and cheese in a medium bowl. Place mixture in the pie crust.
3. **Whisk** together the eggs and half and half in a bowl. Pour the egg mixture over the bacon mixture.
4. **Bake** for 15 minutes. Reduce heat to 350 degrees F (175 degrees C) and bake for 35 minutes more, until top of quiche begins to turn brown.

2. Eggs Benedict with Salmon

Servings: 4
Preparation time: 15 minutes
Cook time: 15 minutes
Ready in: 30 minutes

Nutrition Facts

Serving Size 278 g

Amount Per Serving

Calories 422	Calories from Fat 147

% Daily Value*

Total Fat 16.4g	**25%**
Saturated Fat 4.7g	**23%**
Trans Fat 0.5g	
Cholesterol 523mg	**174%**
Sodium 1701mg	**71%**
Total Carbohydrates 27.3g	**9%**
Dietary Fiber 3.9g	**15%**
Sugars 6.5g	
Protein 34.3g	

Vitamin A 19%	•	Vitamin C 3%
Calcium 21%	•	Iron 21%

Nutrition Grade B-

* Based on a 2000 calorie diet

Ingredients

- 3/4 cup plain low-fat yogurt
- 2 teaspoons white wine
- 2 teaspoons fresh lemon juice
- 3 egg yolks
- 1/2 teaspoon prepared Dijon-style mustard
- 1/4 teaspoon ground cayenne pepper
- 1/4 teaspoon stevia
- 1/4 teaspoon sea salt
- 1 pinch ground black pepper
- 8 (omega-3)eggs
- 8 slices whole wheat bread
- 8 ounces smoked salmon, cut into thin slices
- 2 tablespoons chopped fresh cilantro, for garnish

ections
1. **Whisk** together yogurt, white wine, lemon juice, egg yolks, mustard, cayenne pepper, stevia, salt, and black pepper in a small bowl until light and frothy.
2. **Place** the bowl over a pan of simmering water and whisk constantly for 5 minutes until sauce thickens.
3. **Pour** 8 cups of salted water in a large stock pot and bring to a boil. Carefully break the eggs one at a time into the boiling water. Reduce the heat to medium.
4. **Cook** eggs for about 4 minutes then remove them with a slotted spoon.
5. **Toast** bread slices and place on warm plates. Top each piece of toast with a slice of smoked salmon and a hot poached egg.
6. **Drizzle** with the prepared mustard hollandaise sauce and garnish with cilantro.

3. Zucchini and Beef Breakfast Casserole

Servings: 2
Preparation time: 10 minutes
Cook time: 40 minutes
Ready in: 50 minutes

Nutrition Facts

Serving Size 455 g

Amount Per Serving

Calories 570   Calories from Fat 351

	% Daily Value*
Total Fat 39.0g	60%
Saturated Fat 10.2g	51%
Cholesterol 717mg	239%
Sodium 803mg	33%
Total Carbohydrates 13.8g	5%
Dietary Fiber 3.6g	14%
Sugars 5.4g	
Protein 44.1g	

Vitamin A 26%	•	Vitamin C 43%
Calcium 18%	•	Iron 49%

Nutrition Grade B
* Based on a 2000 calorie diet

Ingredients
- 2 cups lean ground beef

- 4 cloves garlic, minced
- 1 red onion, diced
- 2 tablespoons extra-virgin olive oil, plus extra amount for greasing
- 1 zucchini, peeled and shredded
- 8 eggs
- 2 tablespoons minced fresh thyme
- 3 tablespoon chopped cilantro
- 1/2 teaspoon oregano, chopped
- 1/2 teaspoon sea salt
- 1/4 teaspoon ground black pepper

Directions

1. **Preheat** oven to 350 degrees F. Grease a 9×13 inch baking dish with olive oil.
2. **Place** the ground beef in a medium skillet over medium heat. Stir in the garlic and onion, cook until beef is brown and crumbly. Set aside.
3. **Heat** 2 tablespoons olive oil in another skillet over medium heat. Add the zucchini and cook until tender. Transfer to a bowl and set aside.
4. **Beat** eggs in a large bowl. Stir in the cooked beef, cooked zucchini, thyme, cilantro, oregano, salt, and pepper. Pour mixture into the prepared baking dish.
5. **Cook** in the preheated oven for 30 minutes or until a toothpick inserted into the center comes out clean or with only a few crumbs sticking to it.
6. **Slice** and serve warm.

4. Rosemary Turkey Meatloaf

Servings: 3
Preparation time: 20 minutes
Cook time: 56 minutes
Ready in: 1 hour 16 minutes

Nutrition Facts

Serving Size 326 g

Amount Per Serving

Calories 447 — Calories from Fat 243

	% Daily Value*
Total Fat 27.0g	**42%**
Saturated Fat 6.8g	**34%**
Trans Fat 0.0g	
Cholesterol 219mg	**73%**
Sodium 616mg	**26%**
Total Carbohydrates 20.1g	**7%**
Dietary Fiber 1.6g	**6%**
Sugars 1.8g	
Protein 46.9g	

Vitamin A 16%	•	Vitamin C 48%
Calcium 7%	•	Iron 25%

Nutrition Grade C

* Based on a 2000 calorie diet

Ingredients

- 2 tablespoons extra-virgin olive oil
- 1 clove garlic, chopped
- 1 small onion, chopped
- 1/2 cup red bell pepper, finely chopped
- 1 1/2 pounds lean ground turkey
- 2 tablespoons low-sodium gluten-free Worcestershire sauce
- 1 omega-3 egg, beaten
- 1 tablespoon chopped fresh basil
- 1 tablespoon chopped fresh rosemary
- 1/4 teaspoon sea salt
- 1 teaspoon freshly ground black pepper
- 1/4 cup stevia
- 1 teaspoon water

Directions

1. **Preheat** oven to 350 degrees F (175 degrees C). Line a baking sheet with aluminum foil.

2. **Heat** olive oil in a skillet over medium heat. Add the garlic and sauté until lightly browned. Stir in the onions and red bell pepper; sauté for 5 minutes. Remove from heat and let cool.

3. **Combine** the ground turkey, sautéed onion mixture, 1 tablespoon Worcestershire sauce, egg, basil, rosemary, salt, and pepper.

4. **Shape** turkey mixture into a loaf on the prepared baking sheet. Stir together the stevia, 1 teaspoon of water, and 1 tablespoon Worcestershire sauce in a small bowl. Pour and spread evenly over the top of the loaf.

5. **Bake** for 50 minutes, or until no longer pink in the center and internal temperature reaches 160 degrees F.

6. **Cool** meatloaf for 10 minutes, slice and serve.

5. Veggie Ham Omelet

Servings: 2
Preparation time: 10 minutes
Cook time: 12 minutes
Ready in: 22 minutes

Nutrition Facts

Serving Size 461 g

Amount Per Serving

Calories 570   Calories from Fat 344

	% Daily Value*
Total Fat 38.2g	**59%**
Saturated Fat 18.3g	**92%**
Cholesterol 449mg	**150%**
Sodium 2454mg	**102%**
Total Carbohydrates 17.1g	**6%**
Dietary Fiber 4.2g	**17%**
Sugars 7.2g	
Protein 40.6g	

Vitamin A 26%	•	Vitamin C 63%
Calcium 30%	•	Iron 33%

Nutrition Grade B+

* Based on a 2000 calorie diet

Ingredients

- 2 tablespoons butter
- 1 clove garlic, chopped
- 1 small onion, chopped
- 2 medium red tomatoes, diced
- 1 tablespoon finely chopped fresh jalapeno pepper
- 3/4 cup sliced mushrooms
- 4 eggs
- 2 tablespoons low-fat milk
- 1/2 teaspoon sea salt
- 1 pinch freshly ground black pepper
- 1/2 cup shredded Parmesan cheese
- 8 ounces cooked ham, diced
- 1/2 cup snipped fresh coriander leaves

Directions

1. **Heat** 1 tablespoon of butter in a medium skillet over medium heat. Add garlic and sauté in oil until lightly browned.
2. **Stir** in the onion, tomatoes, jalapeno pepper, and mushrooms; cook for 4 to 5 minutes, stirring occasionally, until vegetables are just tender.
3. **Beat** together the eggs, milk, salt and pepper in a bowl.
4. **Melt** the remaining 1 tablespoon butter in a skillet over medium heat. Coat the skillet with the butter then add the egg mixture and cook for 2 minutes or until partially set. Flip the side with a spatula, and continue cooking 2 to 3 minutes, or until the egg is set.
5. **Sprinkle** the cheese over the omelet and spoon the cooked ham and vegetable mixture into the center.
6. **Fold** omelet over the vegetables and cook for 2 more minutes. Place omelet on a plate, cut in half. Garnish with coriander leaves and serve.

6. No-Crust Cheesy Spinach Quiche

Servings: 3
Preparation time: 15 minutes
Cook time: 30 minutes
Ready in: 45 minutes

Nutrition Facts

Serving Size 346 g

Amount Per Serving

Calories 455   Calories from Fat 267

	% Daily Value*
Total Fat 29.6g	**46%**
Saturated Fat 14.4g	**72%**
Trans Fat 0.0g	
Cholesterol 330mg	**110%**
Sodium 1084mg	**45%**
Total Carbohydrates 13.4g	**4%**
Dietary Fiber 3.8g	**15%**
Sugars 3.5g	
Protein 39.7g	

Vitamin A 201%   •   Vitamin C 59%
Calcium 88%   •   Iron 32%

Nutrition Grade B+
* Based on a 2000 calorie diet

Ingredients
- 1 tablespoon extra-virgin olive oil, plus extra amount for greasing
- 1 onion, chopped
- 1 (10 ounce) package frozen chopped spinach, thawed and drained
- 1 1/2 cup sliced mushrooms
- 5 eggs, beaten
- 4 green onions, chopped
- 3 cups shredded parmesan cheese
- 1/4 teaspoon sea salt
- 1/8 teaspoon ground black pepper
- 1 tablespoon fresh chopped dill

Directions
1. **Preheat** oven to 350 degrees F (175 degrees C). Lightly grease a 9 inch pie pan with olive oil.

2. **Heat** olive oil in a large skillet over medium-high heat. Stir in the onions and cook until translucent. Add the mushrooms and cook for about 6 minutes, or until tender.

3. **Add** the spinach, stir and continue cooking until wilted.

4. **Beat** together the eggs, green onions, cheese, salt, and pepper. Stir in the spinach mixture and blend well. Scoop the mixture into the prepared pie pan.

5. **Bake** for about 30 minutes until eggs have set. Let cool, then slice to serve.

7. Turkey Breakfast Sausage

Servings: 2
Preparation time: 15 minutes
Cook time: 10 minutes
Ready in: 25 minutes

Nutrition Facts

Serving Size 246 g

Amount Per Serving

Calories 610   Calories from Fat 336

	% Daily Value*
Total Fat 37.3g	**57%**
Saturated Fat 8.8g	**44%**
Trans Fat 0.0g	
Cholesterol 231mg	**77%**
Sodium 1181mg	**49%**
Total Carbohydrates 6.0g	**2%**
Dietary Fiber 1.4g	**6%**
Protein 62.7g	

Vitamin A 4%	•	Vitamin C 4%
Calcium 10%	•	Iron 30%

Nutrition Grade B
* Based on a 2000 calorie diet

Ingredients

- 1 teaspoons ground rosemary
- 1 tablespoon Stevia
- 1 teaspoon sea salt
- 1 teaspoon ground black pepper
- 2 cloves garlic, chopped
- 1/4 teaspoon dried oregano
- 1/2 teaspoon ground cayenne pepper
- 1/8 teaspoon nutmeg
- 1 1/2 teaspoon fennel seed
- 1 pound ground turkey
- 1 tablespoon extra-virgin olive oil

Directions

1. **Combine** all ingredients, except the olive oil, in a large bowl.
2. **Shape** mixture into 1/2 inch thick patties.
3. **Grease** a large skillet with the olive oil and place over medium high heat.
4. **Sauté** the patties in the skillet for 5 minutes each side, until no longer pink inside and internal temperature reaches 160 degrees F.

Lunch

8. Spicy Grilled Shrimp

Servings: 6
Preparation time: 40 minutes
Cook time: 12 minutes
Ready in: 52 minutes

Nutrition Facts

Serving Size 298 g

Amount Per Serving

Calories 398	Calories from Fat 149

	% Daily Value*
Total Fat 16.5g	**25%**
Saturated Fat 3.0g	**15%**
Trans Fat 0.0g	
Cholesterol 478mg	**159%**
Sodium 869mg	**36%**
Total Carbohydrates 7.7g	**3%**
Dietary Fiber 0.9g	**4%**
Sugars 1.9g	
Protein 52.3g	

Vitamin A 16%	•	Vitamin C 11%
Calcium 21%	•	Iron 5%

Nutrition Grade B
* Based on a 2000 calorie diet

Ingredients

- 3 cloves garlic, minced
- 1/4 cup extra-virgin olive oil, plus extra amount for greasing
- 1 medium yellow onion, diced
- 1/4 cup organic tomato sauce
- 2 tablespoons white wine vinegar
- 1 tablespoon fresh lemon juice
- 2 tablespoons chopped fresh cilantro
- 1/2 teaspoon sea salt
- 1/4 teaspoon cayenne pepper
- 2 pounds fresh shrimp, peeled and deveined
- Skewers

Directions

1. **Stir** together the garlic, olive oil, onion, tomato sauce, white wine vinegar, lemon juice, cilantro, salt, and cayenne pepper in a large bowl.

2. **Add** shrimp to the bowl, and toss to coat evenly. Cover, and marinate in the fridge for at least 30 minutes, stirring once or twice.

3. **Preheat** grill for medium heat. Thread shrimp onto skewers. Lightly oil grill grate with olive oil.

4. **Grill** shrimp for 2 to 3 minutes per side, or until opaque.

9. Roasted Garlic-Herb Pork

Servings: 3
Preparation time: 15 minutes
Cook time: 30 minutes
Ready in: 45 minutes

Nutrition Facts

Serving Size 254 g

Amount Per Serving

Calories 392	Calories from Fat 121

	% Daily Value*
Total Fat 13.4g	**21%**
Saturated Fat 3.7g	**19%**
Trans Fat 0.1g	
Cholesterol 166mg	**55%**
Sodium 757mg	**32%**
Total Carbohydrates 5.5g	**2%**
Dietary Fiber 2.6g	**10%**
Protein 60.4g	

Vitamin A 12%	•	Vitamin C 14%
Calcium 11%	•	Iron 27%

Nutrition Grade A-
* Based on a 2000 calorie diet

Ingredients

- 1 1/2 pounds boneless lean pork chops
- 4 cloves garlic, peeled and crushed
- 3 tablespoons minced fresh sage
- 1 teaspoon sea salt
- 2 tablespoons chopped oregano

- 1 teaspoon freshly ground black pepper
- 1 teaspoon red pepper flakes
- 1 tablespoon extra-virgin olive oil
- 2 tablespoons fresh lemon juice

Directions
1. **Preheat** oven to 450 degrees F. Place pork in a shallow roasting pan.
2. **Stir** together garlic, sage, salt, oregano, black pepper, red pepper flakes, olive oil, and lemon juice to make a paste.
3. **Rub** garlic paste over all surfaces of pork chops then roast for 15 minutes. Reduce oven temperature down to 300 degrees F.
4. **Roast** 15 to 20 minutes more, or until internal temperature reaches 145 degrees F (63 degrees C). Cool and slice to serve.

10. Salmon Egg Salad

Servings: 3
Ready in: 40 minutes

Nutrition Facts

Serving Size 322 g

Amount Per Serving

Calories 577 — Calories from Fat 348

% Daily Value*

Total Fat 38.7g	**59%**
Saturated Fat 8.0g	**40%**
Trans Fat 0.0g	
Cholesterol 421mg	**140%**
Sodium 839mg	**35%**
Total Carbohydrates 14.9g	**5%**
Dietary Fiber 0.8g	**3%**
Sugars 5.7g	
Protein 41.6g	

Vitamin A 16%	•	Vitamin C 26%
Calcium 10%	•	Iron 15%

Nutrition Grade B

* Based on a 2000 calorie diet

Ingredients
- 14 ounces flaked salmon
- 6 hard-boiled eggs, peeled and chopped
- 1 medium red radish, diced

- 1/2 cup onion, chopped
- 1 1/2 teaspoons Dijon mustard
- 1/2 teaspoon raw honey
- 3/4 cup gluten-free low-fat mayonnaise
- 1/2 sea salt
- 1/8 teaspoon black pepper
- 1/2 teaspoon dried dill
- 2 teaspoons chopped sage
- 1/4 cup chives, chopped

Directions
1. **Place** the salmon, eggs, radish and onions in a large salad bowl.
2. **Stir** together the mustard, honey, mayonnaise, salt, and pepper in a small bowl until combined.
3. **Gently** toss salad with the mayonnaise mixture.
4. **Chill** for at least 30 minutes before serving.

11. Broccoli Fish Bake

Servings: 3
Preparation time: 15 minutes
Cook time: 20 minutes
Ready in: 35 minutes

Nutrition Facts

Serving Size 419 g

Amount Per Serving

Calories 505   Calories from Fat 228

% Daily Value*

Total Fat 25.4g	**39%**
Saturated Fat 12.8g	**64%**
Cholesterol 92mg	**31%**
Sodium 1384mg	**58%**
Total Carbohydrates 19.5g	**6%**
Dietary Fiber 3.8g	**15%**
Sugars 3.3g	
Protein 50.0g	

Vitamin A 33%	•	Vitamin C 65%
Calcium 24%	•	Iron 24%

Nutrition Grade B+
* Based on a 2000 calorie diet

Ingredients

- 1 (10 ounce) package frozen broccoli spears, cooked and drained
- 1 pound fresh halibut fillets
- 1 1/3 cup organic cream of chicken soup
- 1/3 cup coconut milk
- 1/4 cup shredded Cheddar cheese
- 2 tablespoons gluten-free dry bread crumbs
- 1 clove garlic, chopped
- 1/2 teaspoon sea salt
- 1/4 teaspoon ground black pepper
- 1 tablespoon melted butter
- 1/8 teaspoon crushed cayenne pepper flakes

Directions

1. **Preheat** oven to 450 degrees F.
2. **Arrange** broccoli in 2-quart shallow baking dish. Top with the halibut fillets. Mix cream of chicken soup and coconut milk and pour over fish. Sprinkle with cheese.
3. **Combine** the bread crumbs, garlic, salt, pepper, butter, and cayenne pepper; sprinkle mixture on top.
4. **Bake** for 20 minutes or until fish flakes easily with a fork.

12. Grape and Chicken Holiday Salad

Servings: 6
Ready in: 15 minutes

Nutrition Facts

Serving Size 246 g

Amount Per Serving

Calories 531   Calories from Fat 310

	% Daily Value*
Total Fat 34.5g	**53%**
Saturated Fat 5.4g	**27%**
Trans Fat 0.0g	
Cholesterol 98mg	**33%**
Sodium 827mg	**34%**
Total Carbohydrates 24.9g	**8%**
Dietary Fiber 3.0g	**12%**
Sugars 5.9g	
Protein 31.4g	

Vitamin A 13%	•	Vitamin C 22%
Calcium 8%	•	Iron 11%

Nutrition Grade B
* Based on a 2000 calorie diet

Ingredients

- 1 1/2 cup organic low-fat mayonnaise
- 3/4 teaspoon ground cayenne pepper
- 1 teaspoon sea salt
- 1/4 teaspoon ground black pepper
- 1 cup chopped celery
- 2 cups red grapes
- 2 green onions, chopped
- 1/2 cup minced red bell pepper

- 1 cup chopped almonds
- 1 medium red onion, minced
- 4 cups cooked chicken meat, cubed

Directions

1. **Stir** together the mayonnaise, cayenne pepper, salt and black pepper in a medium bowl.
2. **Blend** in celery, red grapes, green onion, bell pepper, almonds, and red onion.
3. **Add** chicken then toss salad with the mayonnaise mixture.
4. **Chill** for 45 minutes before serving.

13. Spicy Turkey & Veggies Stir-Fry

Servings: 3
Preparation time: 15 minutes
Cook time: 35 minutes
Ready in: 50 minutes

Nutrition Facts

Serving Size 520 g

Amount Per Serving

Calories 525　　　　Calories from Fat 270

	% Daily Value*
Total Fat 30.0g	**46%**
Saturated Fat 6.5g	**33%**
Trans Fat 0.0g	
Cholesterol 154mg	**51%**
Sodium 536mg	**22%**
Total Carbohydrates 19.0g	**6%**
Dietary Fiber 5.2g	**21%**
Sugars 9.3g	
Protein 45.2g	

Vitamin A 133%	•	Vitamin C 89%
Calcium 8%	•	Iron 39%

Nutrition Grade B+

* Based on a 2000 calorie diet

Ingredients

- 2 tablespoons olive oil
- 4 cloves garlic, minced
- 1 large onion, chopped
- 1 pound ground turkey

- 1/2 teaspoon dried basil
- 1 teaspoon ground turmeric
- 1/2 teaspoon ground cayenne pepper
- 1/2 teaspoon sea salt
- 1 cup zucchini, diced
- 2 stalks celery, chopped
- 1 cup carrots, diced
- 3 1/2 cups tomatoes, peeled, seeded, and chopped
- 1/2 cup organic low-sodium chicken broth
- 1/2 cup chopped cilantro

Directions

1. **Heat** olive oil in a large pot over medium-high heat.
2. **Add** the garlic and onion, sauté in olive oil for 2 minutes, or until onions are translucent.
3. **Add** ground turkey then stir and cook until no longer pink; season with basil, turmeric, cayenne pepper, and salt.
4. **Stir** in zucchini, celery, carrots, tomatoes, and chicken broth then reduce heat to low.
5. **Simmer** for 25 minutes or until vegetables are tender. Stir in cilantro and serve.

14. Spinach Beef Loaf Muffins

Servings: 4
Preparation time: 15 minutes
Cook time: 30 minutes
Ready in: 45 minutes

Nutrition Facts

Serving Size 273 g

Amount Per Serving

Calories 554 — Calories from Fat 226

% Daily Value*

Total Fat 25.1g	**39%**
Saturated Fat 12.7g	**64%**
Trans Fat 0.0g	
Cholesterol 265mg	**88%**
Sodium 941mg	**39%**
Total Carbohydrates 12.5g	**4%**
Dietary Fiber 0.8g	**3%**
Sugars 2.9g	
Protein 65.3g	

Vitamin A 16% • Vitamin C 5%
Calcium 24% • Iron 181%

Nutrition Grade B

* Based on a 2000 calorie diet

Ingredients

- olive oil for greasing
- 1 1/2 pounds lean ground beef
- 1 1/4 cups crumbled blue cheese
- 2 cloves garlic, crushed and chopped
- 1/2 cup diced onions
- 1/2 cup gluten-free Italian bread crumbs
- 2 eggs
- 1/2 cup chopped fresh spinach
- 1 pinch red pepper flakes
- 2 tablespoons reduced-sodium Worcestershire sauce

Directions

1. **Preheat** oven to 375 degrees F (190 degrees C). Grease a large muffin pan with olive oil.
2. **Mix** all the ingredients in a large bowl until well blended.
3. **Scoop** the meat mixture evenly into the prepared muffin pan.

4. **Bake** for about 30 minutes, or until no longer pink in the center and internal temperature reaches at least 160 degrees F (70 degrees C).

Dinner

15. Herbed Chicken Cordon Bleu

Servings: 6
Preparation time: 15 minutes
Cook time: 40 minutes
Ready in: 55 minutes

Nutrition Facts

Serving Size 278 g

Amount Per Serving

Calories 485	Calories from Fat 233

	% Daily Value*
Total Fat 25.9g	**40%**
Saturated Fat 14.5g	**73%**
Trans Fat 0.0g	
Cholesterol 101mg	**34%**
Sodium 1019mg	**42%**
Total Carbohydrates 17.0g	**6%**
Dietary Fiber 1.5g	**6%**
Sugars 1.9g	
Protein 41.0g	

Vitamin A 24%	Vitamin C 6%
Calcium 28%	Iron 5%

Nutrition Grade D-
* Based on a 2000 calorie diet

Ingredients

- 6 skinless, boneless chicken breast halves, pounded flat
- 6 slices Parmesan cheese
- 6 slices organic ham
- 3 tablespoons gluten-free Panko breadcrumbs
- 1/4 cup fresh chopped basil
- 1 teaspoon paprika
- 2 tablespoons dried rosemary
- 2 tablespoons red pepper flakes
- 6 tablespoons low-fat butter
- 1/2 cup dry white wine
- 1/2 cup melted low-fat butter
- toothpicks

Directions

1. **Lay** a cheese and ham slice on top of each breast. Fold the edges of the chicken over the filling, and secure with toothpicks.

2. **Combine** the breadcrumbs, basil, paprika, rosemary, and red pepper flakes in a small bowl, and coat the chicken pieces.

3. **Heat** the butter in a large skillet over medium-high heat. Add the chicken and cook until evenly browned. Stir in the wine then reduce heat to low.

4. **Cover** and simmer for 30 minutes, until chicken is no longer pink and juices run clear. Discard toothpicks; place the breasts on a serving platter.

5. **Drizzle** with butter and serve warm.

16. Asian Beef Lettuce Wraps

Servings: 3
Preparation time: 15 minutes
Cook time: 15 minutes
Ready in: 30 minutes

Nutrition Facts

Serving Size 352 g

Amount Per Serving

Calories 452	Calories from Fat 164

% **Daily Value***

Total Fat 18.2g	**28%**
Saturated Fat 4.9g	**24%**
Trans Fat 0.0g	
Cholesterol 136mg	**45%**
Sodium 489mg	**20%**
Total Carbohydrates 21.2g	**7%**
Dietary Fiber 3.5g	**14%**
Sugars 10.9g	
Protein 48.9g	

Vitamin A 11%	•	Vitamin C 18%
Calcium 3%	•	Iron 164%

Nutrition Grade A-

* Based on a 2000 calorie diet

Ingredients

- 16 butter lettuce leaves
- 1 pound lean ground beef

- 1 tablespoon extra-virgin olive oil
- 1 large onion, chopped
- 2 cloves fresh garlic, minced
- 1 tablespoon coconut aminos
- 1/4 cup hoisin sauce
- 1 tablespoon minced ginger
- 1 teaspoon red pepper flakes
- 1 tablespoon rice wine vinegar
- 1/2 teaspoon raw honey
- 4 ounce bamboo shoots
- 1 bunch green onions, chopped
- 2 teaspoons sesame oil

Directions

1. **Heat** olive oil in a medium skillet over high heat. Add the ground beef and cook until evenly browned; stirring often. Drain, and transfer to a plate; set aside.
2. **Add** the onion to the same skillet and cook until translucent, stirring frequently. Stir in the garlic, coconut aminos, hoisin sauce, ginger, red pepper flakes, vinegar, and honey.
3. **Stir** in the bamboo shoots, green onions, sesame oil, and cooked beef; cook for about 2 minutes.
4. **Spoon** beef mixture onto lettuce leaves. Roll up and serve.

17. Herbed Pork Chops over Raspberry Sauce

Servings: 3
Preparation time: 15 minutes
Cook time: 18 minutes
Ready in: 33 minutes

Nutrition Facts

Serving Size 227 g

Amount Per Serving

Calories 432   Calories from Fat 168

	% Daily Value*
Total Fat 18.7g	**29%**
Saturated Fat 5.5g	**27%**
Trans Fat 0.1g	
Cholesterol 110mg	**37%**
Sodium 297mg	**12%**
Total Carbohydrates 24.0g	**8%**
Dietary Fiber 2.1g	**8%**
Sugars 14.0g	
Protein 41.5g	

Vitamin A 11%	•	Vitamin C 24%
Calcium 13%	•	Iron 28%

Nutrition Grade B+

* Based on a 2000 calorie diet

Ingredients

- 1/2 teaspoon dried thyme, crushed
- 1/2 teaspoon garlic powder
- 1/2 teaspoon dried sage, crushed
- 1/4 teaspoon sea salt
- 1/4 teaspoon ground black pepper
- 2 tablespoons chopped fresh rosemary
- 2 tablespoons chopped fresh parsley
- 4 (4 ounce) boneless pork loin chops
- 2 tablespoons low-fat butter
- 2 tablespoons olive oil
- 1/4 cup seedless raspberry jam
- 2 tablespoons balsamic vinegar
- 2 tablespoons orange juice
- 4 sprigs fresh dill (optional)

Directions

1. **Preheat** oven to 200 degrees F (95 degrees C).
2. **Mix** together the thyme, garlic powder, sage, salt, pepper, rosemary, and parsley. Rub evenly over pork chops.
3. **Melt** butter and olive oil in a skillet over medium heat. Add the seasoned pork chops and cook for 4 to 5 minutes on each side, turning once.
4. **Remove** from skillet and keep warm in preheated oven.
5. **Stir** together the raspberry jam, vinegar, and orange juice. Bring to a boil, and cook for 2 to 3 minutes, until sauce is thick or desired consistency is reached.
6. **Spoon** sauce plate, and top with pork chops. Garnish with sprigs of dill.

18. Cajun Chicken Jambalaya

Servings: 4
Preparation time: 15 minutes
Cook time: 30 minutes
Ready in: 45 minutes

Nutrition Facts

Serving Size 603 g

Amount Per Serving

Calories 548   Calories from Fat 187

	% Daily Value*
Total Fat 20.8g	**32%**
Saturated Fat 6.3g	**31%**
Trans Fat 0.0g	
Cholesterol 346mg	**115%**
Sodium 1142mg	**48%**
Total Carbohydrates 21.1g	**7%**
Dietary Fiber 6.0g	**24%**
Sugars 10.0g	
Protein 68.7g	

Vitamin A 100%	•	Vitamin C 235%
Calcium 13%	•	Iron 44%

Nutrition Grade B+

* Based on a 2000 calorie diet

Ingredients

- 2 tablespoon butter
- 1 tablespoon olive oil

- 1 large onion, diced
- 2 Linguica sausage, halved lengthwise and cut into 1/4-inch half-moons
- 6 cloves garlic, finely chopped
- 3 green bell peppers, seeded and diced
- 1 3/4 cup crushed fresh tomatoes
- 1 zucchini, diced
- 1 tablespoon paprika
- 1/2 tablespoon dried oregano
- 1/2 tablespoon cayenne pepper
- 1 teaspoon hot sauce
- 1 cup low-sodium chicken broth
- 1 pound chicken breast, cooked, cooled, and chopped
- 1 pound cooked, peeled, and deveined shrimp

Directions

1. **Heat** the butter and olive oil in a large saucepan over medium heat.
2. **Stir** in the onion and sausage and cook for 10 minutes, or until the onion starts to brown. Add the garlic and stir and cook for about 2 minutes until fragrant.
3. **Stir** in green bell peppers, tomatoes, zucchinis, paprika, oregano, cayenne pepper, hot sauce, and chicken broth.
4. **Bring** mixture to a boil then reduce to a simmer. Cook uncovered for about 15 minutes until the mixture is thick.
5. **Add** the chicken and shrimp, stir and simmer for about 2 minutes until heated through.

19. Spinach and Mushroom Stuffed Chicken

Servings: 6
Preparation time: 15 minutes
Cook time: 1 hour
Ready in: 1 hour and 15 minutes

Nutrition Facts

Serving Size 408 g

Amount Per Serving

Calories 543 — Calories from Fat 190

% Daily Value*

Total Fat 21.2g	**33%**
Saturated Fat 5.9g	**30%**
Trans Fat 0.0g	
Cholesterol 34mg	**11%**
Sodium 757mg	**32%**
Total Carbohydrates 18.0g	**6%**
Dietary Fiber 2.5g	**10%**
Sugars 5.6g	
Protein 70.0g	

Vitamin A 94%	Vitamin C 31%
Calcium 17%	Iron 15%

Nutrition Grade B
* Based on a 2000 calorie diet

Ingredients

- 3/4 cup mayonnaise
- 1 onion, chopped
- 1 (10 ounce) package frozen chopped spinach, thawed and drained
- 1 teaspoon chopped fresh oregano
- 1 cup sliced mushrooms
- 1/2 cup crumbled Monterey jack cheese
- 3/4 cup sundried tomatoes
- 2 cloves garlic, chopped
- 1/2 teaspoon dried basil
- 4 skinless, boneless chicken breasts, butterflied
- 4 slices bacon

Directions

1. **Preheat** oven to 375 degrees F (190 degrees C).
2. **Combine** the mayonnaise, onion, spinach, oregano, mushrooms, cheese, tomatoes, garlic, and basil in a medium bowl. Blend well and set aside.
3. **Spoon** the prepared spinach mixture into the butterflied chicken breasts. Wrap each with a piece of bacon, and secure with a toothpick then place in shallow baking dish and cover.
4. **Bake** for 1 hour, or until chicken is no longer pink in the center and the internal temperature reaches at least 165 degrees F (74 degrees C).
5. **Let** cool slightly, then slice and serve.

20. Herb Crusted Cod Fillets

Servings: 2
Preparation time: 10 minutes
Cook time: 10 minutes
Ready in: 20 minutes

Nutrition Facts

Serving Size 387 g

Amount Per Serving

Calories 490	Calories from Fat 192

	% Daily Value*
Total Fat 21.4g	**33%**
Saturated Fat 2.5g	**13%**
Trans Fat 0.0g	
Cholesterol 167mg	**56%**
Sodium 702mg	**29%**
Total Carbohydrates 10.6g	**4%**
Dietary Fiber 5.2g	**21%**
Sugars 1.4g	
Protein 65.1g	

Vitamin A 14%	•	Vitamin C 21%
Calcium 10%	•	Iron 12%

Nutrition Grade C+
* Based on a 2000 calorie diet

Ingredients

- 4 (6 oz.) skinless cod fillets
- 2 tablespoon extra-virgin olive oil
- 2 tablespoons mustard

- 2 tablespoon coconut flour
- 4 tablespoons fresh flat-leaf cilantro, chopped
- 2 cloves garlic, crushed
- 1 tablespoon fresh rosemary, chopped
- 1/2 teaspoon sea salt
- 1/4 ground black pepper

Directions

1. **Preheat** oven to 450 degrees. Line a baking sheet with parchment paper or foil.
2. **Stir** together the olive oil and mustard in a small bowl and rub into the fish. Place fish into the prepared baking sheet.
3. **Mix** the coconut flour, cilantro, garlic, rosemary, and salt and pepper in another bowl.
4. **Spoon** the prepared herb mixture on top of the fish fillets, pressing down on each.
5. **Bake** in the preheated oven for 10-15 minutes or until fish flakes easily with a fork.

21. Spaghetti Squash with Garlic Meat Sauce

Servings: 6
Preparation time: 15 minutes
Cook time: 1 hour
Ready in: 1 hour and 15 minutes

Nutrition Facts

Serving Size 362 g

Amount Per Serving

Calories 377	Calories from Fat 89

	% Daily Value*
Total Fat 9.9g	**15%**
Saturated Fat 3.6g	**18%**
Cholesterol 135mg	**45%**
Sodium 330mg	**14%**
Total Carbohydrates 21.1g	**7%**
Dietary Fiber 4.6g	**18%**
Sugars 11.6g	
Protein 50.5g	

Vitamin A 24%	Vitamin C 61%
Calcium 5%	Iron 179%

Nutrition Grade A

* Based on a 2000 calorie diet

Ingredients

- 1 (2 pounds) spaghetti squash, halved lengthwise and seeded
- 1 medium head of garlic, cloves crushed
- 2 pounds ground beef
- 1 medium onion, chopped
- 1 1/2 cup organic tomato paste
- 1 cup shredded fresh basil leaves, plus extra amount for garnish
- 4 sun-dried tomatoes, diced
- 1/2 teaspoon sea salt
- 1/4 teaspoon ground black pepper
- olive oil for greasing

Directions

1. **Preheat** oven to 350 degrees F. Grease a roasting pan with olive oil.

2. **Place** the squash halves with cut sides down in the prepared roasting pan. Roast in the oven for about 30-45 minutes until tender.
3. **Meanwhile**, place a skillet over medium-high heat. Add the garlic and sauté until lightly browned.
4. **Stir** in the ground beef and onion, cook until evenly browned. Add the tomato paste, basil, sun-dried tomatoes, salt, and pepper.
5. **Reduce** heat to medium and simmer for 20 minutes.
6. **Remove** roasted squash from oven and let cool slightly. Scrape the inside of the roasted spaghetti squash halves with a fork and divide onto plates.
7. **Pour** cooked meat sauce over the top, and sprinkle with basil.

22. Cherry Cheesecake Bars

Servings: 4
Preparation time: 10 minutes
Cook time: 42 minutes
Ready in: 52 minutes

Nutrition Facts

Serving Size 132 g

Amount Per Serving

Calories 340	Calories from Fat 239

% Daily Value*

Total Fat 26.6g	**41%**
Saturated Fat 6.2g	**31%**
Trans Fat 0.0g	
Cholesterol 62mg	**21%**
Sodium 219mg	**9%**
Total Carbohydrates 28.7g	**10%**
Dietary Fiber 2.5g	**10%**
Sugars 10.5g	
Protein 10.7g	

Vitamin A 2%	•	Vitamin C 4%
Calcium 4%	•	Iron 7%

Nutrition Grade D

* Based on a 2000 calorie diet

Ingredients

- 1/4 cup low-fat butter, softened
- 1/4 cup stevia
- 1 teaspoon ground cinnamon
- 1 cup almond flour
- 1/4 cup walnuts, chopped
- 100 g low-fat sugar-free cream cheese, softened
- 1 omega-3 egg
- 2 tablespoons coconut milk
- 1 teaspoon pure vanilla extract
- 1/4 cup organic cherry jam

Directions

1. **Preheat** oven to 350 degrees F (175 degrees C).

2. **Combine** and stir together the butter, stevia, cinnamon, flour, and walnuts stir until mixture becomes crumbly.

3. **Press** 3/4 cup of pastry mixture into 8-inch square baking pan. Set aside remaining pastry mixture.

4. **Bake** for 12 to 15 minutes then cool crust on a wire rack.

5. **Whisk** together the cream cheese, egg, coconut milk, and vanilla. Swirl cherry jam through the filling.

6. **Spread** cream cheese mixture over baked crust. Sprinkle reserved pastry mixture on as a topping.

7. **Bake** for about 30 minutes. Let cool on wire rack. Cover and chill in the fridge. Slice to serve.

23. Carrot Banana Muffins

Servings: 5
Preparation time: 15 minutes
Cook time: 20 minutes
Ready in: 35 minutes

Nutrition Facts

Serving Size 125 g

Amount Per Serving

Calories 434	Calories from Fat 313

	% Daily Value*
Total Fat 34.8g	**54%**
Saturated Fat 20.5g	**103%**
Trans Fat 0.0g	
Cholesterol 98mg	**33%**
Sodium 369mg	**15%**
Total Carbohydrates 20.7g	**7%**
Dietary Fiber 4.8g	**19%**
Sugars 13.0g	
Protein 14.1g	

Vitamin A 76%	•	Vitamin C 6%
Calcium 8%	•	Iron 14%

Nutrition Grade C-

* Based on a 2000 calorie diet

Ingredients
- 3 eggs
- 1/2 cup raw honey
- 1/2 cup coconut oil, melted
- 1 tablespoon pure vanilla extract

- 1/2 teaspoon baking soda
- 1/2 teaspoon sea salt
- 2 teaspoons cinnamon
- 1 cup soy flour
- 1 cup shredded carrots
- 1 cup chopped hazelnuts
- 1/2 cup chopped dried cranberries

Directions

1. **Preheat** oven to 350 degrees F. Line a 12-cup muffin tin with muffin liners.
2. **Beat** together the eggs, honey, coconut oil, and vanilla in a large mixing bowl. Add the baking soda, salt, cinnamon, and flour; whisk until smooth.
3. **Fold** in the shredded carrots, hazelnuts, and dried cranberries; stir to combine. Scoop the batter evenly into the prepared muffin cups.
4. **Bake** for 20 minutes, or until a toothpick inserted into the center of the muffin comes out clean or with only a few crumbs sticking to it.

24. Fresh Fruit Salad with Lemon Coconut Cream

Servings: 3
Ready in: 20 minutes

Nutrition Facts

Serving Size 249 g

Amount Per Serving

Calories 389	Calories from Fat 254

	% Daily Value*
Total Fat 28.3g	**43%**
Saturated Fat 9.9g	**50%**
Cholesterol 0mg	**0%**
Sodium 50mg	**2%**
Total Carbohydrates 27.6g	**9%**
Dietary Fiber 8.1g	**33%**
Sugars 14.9g	
Protein 10.3g	

Vitamin A 6%	•	Vitamin C 76%
Calcium 16%	•	Iron 17%

Nutrition Grade B+

* Based on a 2000 calorie diet

Ingredients

- 1 peach, pitted and sliced
- 1 cup sliced strawberries
- 1 cup fresh blueberries
- 1 cup chopped hazelnuts
- 2 tablespoons freshly squeezed lemon juice
- 1/2 cup coconut cream
- 1 cup natural soy milk
- 2 tablespoons ground flax seeds
- 1/4 cup rolled oats

Directions

1. **Combine** peach, strawberries, blueberries, and hazelnuts in a large salad bowl.
2. **Stir** together lemon juice, coconut cream, and soy milk then pour over salad.
3. **Sprinkle** with ground flax seeds and oats, gently toss to coat.
4. **Chill** and serve.

25. Avocado Hazelnut Mousse

Servings: 3
Ready in: 15 minutes

Nutrition Facts

Serving Size 200 g

Amount Per Serving

Calories 456	Calories from Fat 336

% Daily Value*

Total Fat 37.3g	**57%**
Saturated Fat 3.5g	**17%**
Trans Fat 0.0g	
Cholesterol 0mg	**0%**
Sodium 39mg	**2%**
Total Carbohydrates 21.5g	**7%**
Dietary Fiber 13.1g	**52%**
Sugars 9.5g	
Protein 12.3g	

Vitamin A 2%	•	Vitamin C 15%
Calcium 12%	•	Iron 17%

Nutrition Grade C+

* Based on a 2000 calorie diet

Ingredients

- 1 avocado, peeled and pitted
- 1 cup organic soy milk
- 1 tablespoon organic maple syrup
- 1/2 teaspoon pure vanilla extract
- 1 1/2 cups chopped hazelnuts
- 1/4 cup flax seeds

Directions

1. **Place** all ingredients in a food processor and process until smooth.
2. **Chill** for about 20 minutes before serving.

26. Low Carb Granola Snack

Servings: 6
Preparation time: 10 minutes
Cook time: 20 minutes
Ready in: 30 minutes

Nutrition Facts

Serving Size 107 g

Amount Per Serving

Calories 456 — Calories from Fat 296

	% Daily Value*
Total Fat 32.9g	**51%**
Saturated Fat 10.1g	**50%**
Trans Fat 0.0g	
Cholesterol 0mg	**0%**
Sodium 10mg	**0%**
Total Carbohydrates 27.5g	**9%**
Dietary Fiber 14.7g	**59%**
Sugars 14.2g	
Protein 12.0g	

Vitamin A 5%	•	Vitamin C 5%	
Calcium 10%	•	Iron 15%	

Nutrition Grade C-

* Based on a 2000 calorie diet

Ingredients

- 1 cups rolled oats
- 1 cup chopped pecans
- 1/2 cup raw sunflower seeds
- 1/4 cup coconut oil
- 1/4 cup raw honey
- 1 tablespoon ground cinnamon
- 1 teaspoon pure vanilla extract
- 1/2 cup chopped dried apricot
- 1/2 cup dried cranberries
- 1 cup flax seeds

Directions

1. **Preheat** oven to 300 degrees F (150 degrees C).
2. **Mix** together the oats, pecans, and sunflower seeds in a large bowl. Stir together the coconut oil, honey, cinnamon, and

vanilla then pour mixture over dry ingredients; stir to combine.

3. **Spread** mixture onto two ungreased baking sheets.
4. **Bake** for 20 minutes, stirring occasionally.
5. **Let** cool, and then stir in the dried apricots, cranberries, and flax seeds. Store in an airtight container.

27. Creamy Peanut Butter Balls

Servings: 6
Ready in: 1 hour and 15 minutes

Nutrition Facts

Serving Size 126 g

Amount Per Serving

Calories 509   Calories from Fat 332

% **Daily Value***

Total Fat 36.9g	**57%**
Saturated Fat 7.3g	**37%**
Trans Fat 0.0g	
Cholesterol 6mg	**2%**
Sodium 307mg	**13%**
Total Carbohydrates 24.2g	**8%**
Dietary Fiber 10.6g	**42%**
Sugars 12.5g	
Protein 24.4g	

Vitamin A 1%	•	Vitamin C 6%
Calcium 9%	•	Iron 11%

Nutrition Grade C

* Based on a 2000 calorie diet

Ingredients
- 1 1/2 cups organic crunchy peanut butter
- 2 scoops cocoa whey protein powder
- 2 teaspoons ground cinnamon
- 2 ripe bananas, mashed
- 2 teaspoons pure vanilla extract
- 1/2 cups flax seeds

Directions
1. **Combine** all the ingredients in a large bowl.
2. **Mold** the mixture into 1/2 inch balls, and place in a shallow container.

3. **Freeze** for at least 1 hour before serving.

28. Mixed Berries Parfait

Servings: 6
Ready in: 15 minutes

Nutrition Facts

Serving Size 126 g

Amount Per Serving

Calories 461　　　　Calories from Fat 335

% Daily Value*

Total Fat 37.2g	**57%**
Saturated Fat 22.5g	**112%**
Trans Fat 0.0g	
Cholesterol 0mg	**0%**
Sodium 6mg	**0%**
Total Carbohydrates 21.9g	**7%**
Dietary Fiber 16.7g	**67%**
Sugars 11.6g	
Protein 10.1g	

Vitamin A 1%	•	Vitamin C 33%
Calcium 8%	•	Iron 17%

Nutrition Grade B-

* Based on a 2000 calorie diet

Ingredients

- 1 cup fresh blueberries
- 1 cup sliced fresh strawberries
- 1 cup melted coconut butter
- 2 tablespoons agave nectar
- 1 cup chopped hazelnuts
- 3/4 cup flax seeds
- 1 tablespoon chopped fresh mint

Directions

1. **Place** the berries into parfait glasses.
2. **Stir** together the coconut butter and agave nectar in a small bowl until smooth.
3. **Pour** half of the coconut butter mixture over the berries.
4. **Add** the chopped hazelnuts and flax seeds over the top. Pour in the remaining coconut butter mixture.
5. **Sprinkle** fresh mint on top. Chill before serving.

Books by Maggie Fitzgerald

The 7-Day Acid Reflux Diet

The 3-Step Diabetic Diet Plan

The Anti-Inflammatory Diet Plan

Ketogenic Diet Crash Course

Atkins Diet Beginners' Crash Course

www.amazon.com/author/robertfleischer

About Robert M. Fleischer

Besides being a noted author, Robert M. Fleischer is a California-based health researcher, husband and a father of 2 children, one boy and one girl. He has dedicated his career to developing better standards of care and treatment for patients of common, chronic and misunderstood conditions which are often handled with pharmaceuticals to treat the symptoms rather than lifestyle changes which address the root cause.

In his spare time he enjoys tennis, mountain biking and is a member of a local amateur theater group.

Exclusive Bonus Download: All You Wanted To Know About The Raw Food Diet

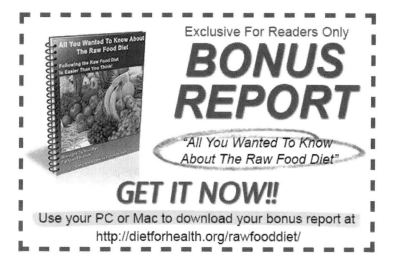

Download your bonus, please visit the download link above from your PC or MAC. To open PDF files, visit http://get.adobe.com/reader/ to download the reader if it's not already installed on your PC or Mac. To open ZIP files, you may need to download WinZip from http://www.winzip.com. This download is for PC or Mac ONLY and might not be downloadable to kindle.

Raw food diets can be a great way to not only lose weight but also led a much healthier, natural lifestyle in general. Most raw food diets are plant-based, with at least 75% of the diet composed of raw food.

This short report will give you a bird's eye view about this all-natural diet plan!

You will learn:

- What is The Raw Food Diet Really Is!
- The Pros and Cons of the Rww Food Diet!
- Tools of the Trade!
- 7 Simple and Easy Raw Food Diet Meal Plans
- And MUCH MUCH MORE!

Visit the URL above to download this guide and start improving your health NOW

One Last Thing...

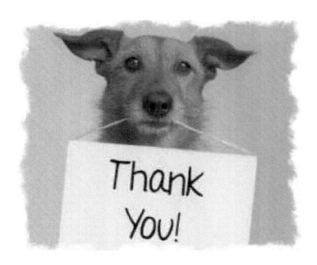

Thank you so much for reading my book. I hope you really liked it. As you probably know, many people look at the reviews on Amazon before they decide to purchase a book. If you liked the book, could you please take a minute to leave a review with your feedback? 60 seconds is all I'm asking for, and it would mean the world to me.

Robert M. Fleischer

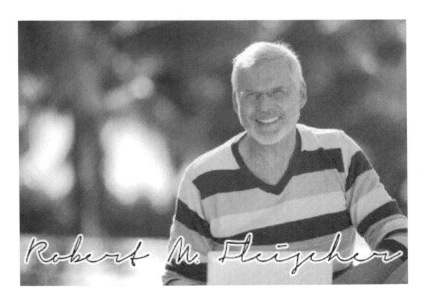

Copyright © 2012 Robert M. Fleischer

Images and Cover by NaturalWay Publishing

NaturalWay
Publishing

Atlanta, Georgia USA